Panic Disorder and Anxiety
in Adolescence

Parent, Adolescent and Child Training Skills 2
Series Editor: Martin Herbert

Panic Disorder and Anxiety
in Adolescence

by

Sara G. Mattis and Thomas H. Ollendick

Series Editor
Martin Herbert

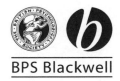

BPS Blackwell

Editorial Offices:
108 Cowley Road, Oxford OX4 1JF, UK
    Tel: +44 (0)1865 791100
350 Main Street, Malden, MA 02148-5018, USA
    Tel: +1 781 388 8250

First published 2002 by The British Psychological Society and Blackwell Publishers Ltd,
a Blackwell Publishing company

Library of Congress Cataloging-in-Publication Data has been applied for

ISBN 1 85433 352 6 (paperback)

A catalogue record for this title is available from the British Library.

Set in Lapidary
by Ralph J. Footring, Derby
Printed and bound in Great Britain
by T J International, Padstow, Cornwall

For further information on
Blackwell Publishers, visit our website:
www.blackwellpublishers.co.uk

Contents

Panic disorder and anxiety in adolescence

Introduction

Adolescence is a developmental period characterized by vast physical, cognitive, social and emotional changes. This time of life marks a progression towards independence as new social contacts beyond the immediate family are established and consolidated, and individual goals and aspirations take centre stage. For some, however, problems with panic and anxiety may manifest themselves during adolescence, causing significant distress and interfering in the critical developmental tasks of this period. Fortunately, much new knowledge has been gained regarding the nature and treatment of panic and other anxiety disorders during adolescence.

Aims

The purpose of this guide is to convey some of this knowledge to counsellors, school personnel, doctors, nurses, psychologists, social workers and other professionals who work with adolescents, with the goal of improving quality of life during this important developmental period.

Objectives

After reading this guide, practitioners should have a greater understanding of:

➢ the nature and characteristics of panic and anxiety in adolescents;
➢ the three components of anxiety and the ways in which they are manifested during adolescence;
➢ the causes of panic in adolescence;
➢ assessment strategies useful in understanding an adolescent's anxiety;
➢ treatment approaches that may help adolescents learn to cope with anxiety, decrease avoidance and improve quality of life;
➢ the ways in which parents may assist teens in overcoming difficulties with anxiety;
➢ special issues that should be considered in working with adolescents with anxiety.

Part I: Panic in adolescents

Although controversy has existed regarding the extent to which panic attacks and panic disorder occur in children and adolescents, many clinical researchers and practitioners now agree that panic not only exists before adulthood, but that it often begins during adolescence (Bernstein *et al.*, 1996). Indeed, 40–60 per cent of teenagers report panic attacks, while approximately one out of every 100 teenagers experiences panic disorder, a disorder characterized by sudden, unexpected rushes of intense anxiety (for review, see Ollendick *et al.*, 1994). Panic is thus a relatively common yet frequently misunderstood experience of adolescence.

What are panic attacks?

A panic attack is defined in the fourth edition of the *Diagnostic and Statistical Manual of Mental Disorders* (DSM-IV; American Psychiatric Association, 1994) as a sudden episode of intense fear, apprehension, or discomfort which is accompanied by at least four of the following physical or cognitive symptoms increasing in intensity within 10 minutes (attacks having fewer than four symptoms are designated as 'limited-symptom attacks'):

- ➤ palpitations/pounding heart;
- ➤ sweating;
- ➤ trembling or shaking;
- ➤ sensations of shortness of breath or smothering;
- ➤ feeling of choking;
- ➤ chest pain or discomfort;
- ➤ nausea or abdominal distress;
- ➤ dizziness or light-headedness
- ➤ derealization or depersonalisation;
- ➤ numbness or tingling sensations;
- ➤ chills or hot flushes;
- ➤ fear of losing control or going crazy;
- ➤ fear of dying.

Three types of panic attacks have been identified:

- ➤ *unexpected or uncued panic attacks* are not associated with a situational trigger and thus occur spontaneously or 'out of the blue';

➤ *situationally-bound or cued panic attacks* almost always occur immediately upon exposure to, or in anticipation of, a situational trigger (e.g. a teenager experiences a panic attack every time she is called on to speak in front of the class);

➤ *situationally-predisposed panic attacks* are more likely to occur upon exposure to a situational cue, but do not always occur immediately upon exposure (e.g. a teenager is more likely to have a panic attack in a cinema, but he does not always have a panic attack in this situation or he may experience a panic attack an hour into the film).

These three types of panic attack may occur across a variety of anxiety disorders. An adolescent must experience recurrent unexpected panic attacks to receive a diagnosis of panic disorder, although situationally-predisposed panic attacks are also common in this disorder. Situationally-bound panic attacks are most typical of social and specific phobias. Some adolescents may experience occasional panic attacks in the absence of an anxiety disorder.

In most cases, however, adolescents experiencing a panic attack describe feelings of impending doom and an intense desire to escape.

Non-clinical panic attacks

Non-clinical panic attacks are those that occur in individuals who are not seeking treatment (Norton *et al.*, 1986). They appear to be a fairly common experience of adolescence. Recent research has examined the prevalence and characteristics of non-clinical panic by asking teenagers to complete questionnaires or interviews regarding their experiences with panic (for review, see Ollendick *et al.*, 1994). The following conclusions can be drawn from this research:

➤ panic is a relatively common experience of adolescence (36–63 per cent of adolescent community samples report panic attacks);
➤ girls report experiencing more panic attacks than boys;
➤ American adolescents report slightly more panic attacks than Australian adolescents;
➤ the frequency and severity of panic attacks are directly related to anxiety, depression and stress, and are inversely related to social support.

Prevalence of panic attacks and symptoms

King *et al.* (1993, 1996) have conducted two studies aimed at investigating panic attacks in Australian adolescents. In each study, adolescents were asked to complete a panic attack questionnaire which included questions pertaining to frequency of panic attacks and associated symptoms, as well as to situations in which panic had occurred. The first study examined 246 13 to 15-year-olds and 288 16 to 18-year-olds. Of the entire sample, 43 per cent reported experiencing a panic attack at some point in their lives, although most experienced only a few symptoms (e.g. limited symptom attacks). The most common symptoms were:

➢ pounding heart (endorsed by 71 per cent of panickers);
➢ trembling or shaking (53 per cent);
➢ sweating (38 per cent);
➢ nausea (34 per cent).

Of the cognitive symptoms, *fear of dying* was reported by 17 per cent of the adolescents with panic attacks, while 19 per cent reported *fear of going crazy or doing something uncontrolled* during an attack.

A greater proportion of females (47 per cent) than males (39 per cent) reported panic attacks. While most adolescents perceived their panic attacks as causing little interference in their lives, approximately 7 per cent reported notable interference. Indeed, 25 per cent reported *avoidance* of particular situations (e.g. giving a speech, being alone at night, going to the hospital) owing to fear of having a panic attack. Finally, adolescent panickers reported significantly more general anxiety than their peers who had never experienced a panic attack, which suggests that highly anxious adolescents may be at risk for the development of panic.

In a second similar study, King *et al.* (1996) found that 36 per cent of 649 Australian adolescents (aged 12–17) reported experiencing a panic attack at some point in their lives, although only 16 per cent reported full-blown panic attacks meeting DSM-IV criteria (see above). Females were more likely than males to report such full-blown attacks (66 per cent vs 34 per cent). The most frequently endorsed symptoms were:

➢ trembling (86 per cent);
➢ dizziness or faintness (80 per cent);
➢ pounding heart (79 per cent);
➢ sweating (75 per cent).

The most common situations associated with panic attacks were:

➢ separation from someone important (42 per cent);
➢ walking alone at night (39 per cent);
➢ tests (38 per cent);
➢ being watched or stared at (37 per cent).

Unexpected panic attacks were reported by 21 per cent of adolescent panickers. Finally, adolescents who had experienced panic attacks reported higher levels of general anxiety, depression and fear than did non-panickers. Family factors also played an important role, with adolescent panickers reporting less family support and more family-associated stress and pressure compared with their peers who had never experienced a panic attack. It is important for professionals who work with teenagers to be tuned into such risk factors and the role they may play in the development of panic attacks during adolescence.

What is panic disorder?

Adolescents with panic disorder experience recurrent, unexpected panic attacks followed by at least one month of persistent concern about having additional attacks, worry about the implications or consequences of the attacks, or a significant change in behaviour related to the attacks. For instance, a teenager with panic disorder may worry that she is losing control or 'going crazy', or she may believe that the physical symptoms of the panic attacks are the result of a serious illness.

Many teenagers with panic disorder develop *agoraphobia*, defined as anxiety about being in situations from which escape might be difficult (or embarrassing) or help might not be readily available if the sufferer were to experience a panic attack. Adolescents with agoraphobia typically avoid such situations, or will enter them only with a 'safe person', such as a parent. Indeed, many adolescents with panic disorder begin to avoid a variety of situations, such as cinemas, classrooms, stores, public transport and being alone, for fear of having a panic attack.

According to DSM-IV, there is much variability in the age at onset of panic disorder, although it typically begins between late adolescence and the mid-30s (although several cases have their onset in childhood). There is some suggestion that late adolescence is the initial peak for the onset of panic disorder, which emphasizes how important it is that adults working with teenagers be aware of warning signs suggesting the development of panic disorder during adolescence.

A brief screening instrument for determining the possible presence of panic attacks and panic disorder in adolescents is provided in Appendix 1. Following is a case description of a young adolescent suffering from panic disorder with agoraphobia:

> Beth was 13 years old when she came with her mother to receive an assessment for anxiety. Her mother reported concern regarding Beth's complaints of physical symptoms (e.g. dizziness, light-headedness) as well as anxiety surrounding going to school and separating from her. These difficulties reportedly followed an episode

during which Beth experienced intense anxiety and several physical symptoms (e.g. difficulty breathing, light-headedness) while in a cinema with her mother and a friend approximately four months before the assessment. During this episode, Beth reported that she had suddenly felt very scared for no reason and that she felt as if she could not take deep breaths and her throat was closing and tightening. As a result of this episode, Beth's mother had taken her to a local hospital, where she underwent several food allergy tests, all of which were negative.

Beth acknowledged that she sometimes felt very scared out of the blue, and that these feelings of fear were associated with certain physical sensations (e.g. light-headedness, butterflies in her stomach). After the initial incident in the cinema, Beth reported that she had a similar episode the next day while at home, and that the episodes had continued erratically, occurring a total of five to ten times, with two to five occurring in the past month. Beth endorsed several physical symptoms associated with these episodes of anxiety, including a pounding heart, difficulty breathing, feeling of choking, chest pain or discomfort, butterflies in her stomach, dizziness and light-headedness, and tingling in her hands. She also reported that she worried about having additional anxiety episodes, particularly at school, and that she was afraid she would 'pass out or have trouble breathing again'.

Finally, Beth reported avoidance of certain situations due to fear that she would have such an anxiety episode and would not be able to get out of the situation or get help. Specifically, she reported that she had not gone to a cinema since the initial episode, and that she was afraid of taking the bus to school for fear that the driver would not know what to do if she suddenly felt anxious. Other situations she endorsed as the focus of fear or avoidance were classrooms, school dances, public transport and church. Beth's mother reported that Beth would sometimes want to leave certain situations (e.g. shopping, a soccer game) due to these feelings of anxiety, and that her presence seemed to help reduce Beth's anxiety in some situations (e.g. shops or malls). Both Beth and her mother were very concerned about the amount of interference Beth's anxiety was causing in her life and her relationships. Beth was diagnosed with panic disorder with agoraphobia.

Part II: Other anxiety disorders associated with panic in adolescents

While panic disorder and its associated avoidance can be particularly debilitating for adolescents, other types of anxiety can also cause considerable distress and interference in an individual's life during the teenage years. These other anxiety disorders frequently coexist with panic disorder in adolescence, and panic attacks, as described above, may occur within any of them.

> *Social phobia* seriously impairs a teenager's ability to participate in social activities that are critical components of adolescence, including going to parties and school dances with friends, meeting new people and dating.
> *Obsessive-compulsive disorder* may lock teenagers into a lonely world where they feel captive to intrusive thoughts and rituals that are often difficult to understand and discuss with peers.
> Adolescents suffering from *generalized anxiety disorder* experience uncontrollable worry that may lead to difficulty relaxing and irritability, again causing significant distress and interfering in relationships.
> *Specific phobias* may lead an adolescent to avoid certain feared situations, such as dogs, heights or airplanes, again limiting activities (e.g. a teenager with a specific phobia of flying may be unable to join an important school or club trip). These other anxiety disorders that impact the lives of adolescents are described below.

Social phobia

Social phobia in adolescents is characterized by considerable anxiety in and avoidance of social or performance situations (e.g. dating, parties, school presentations) due to fears of rejection or negative evaluation. When faced with a feared situation, teenagers with social phobia will almost always experience immediate anxiety, which may take the form of a *situationally-bound or situationally-predisposed panic attack* (see above). Symptoms that are typically experienced in social or performance situations include a pounding heart, trembling, sweating, stomach distress and blushing.

Adolescents with social phobia often experience intense embarrassment and fear that others will think they appear anxious, 'weird', or stupid. When speaking in front of others or having a conversation, they may worry that their anxiety will appear obvious, with others noticing that they are shaking or having difficulty expressing themselves. Even basic activities such as eating, drinking or writing in public may be avoided because of fear of embarrassment. Social phobia typically begins in the mid-teens, causes significant distress and interferes in daily activities and social relationships.

Obsessive-compulsive disorder

The presence of recurrent *obsessions* or *compulsions* is the primary feature of *obsessive-compulsive disorder*. Obsessions are persistent and intrusive thoughts or impulses which cause notable anxiety. Common obsessions experienced by adolescents with obsessive-compulsive disorder include persistent thoughts about contamination (e.g. being contaminated by germs on doorknobs or in the school toilets), recurrent doubts about one's actions (e.g. did I run over someone while I was driving?), needing to keep things in a certain order (e.g. books and other items may need to be arranged in a specific and rigid manner in a locker), horrific or aggressive impulses (e.g. to hurt a parent or shout an obscenity in class) and distressing sexual imagery (e.g. a persistent pornographic image). An adolescent experiencing obsessions will typically try to ignore the thoughts or to neutralize them with another thought or action (i.e. a compulsion).

Compulsions are repetitive actions a person performs with the goal of preventing or reducing feelings of anxiety. Adolescents with obsessive-compulsive disorder often feel driven to perform certain compulsions to reduce the distress caused by an obsession or to prevent a dreaded consequence. For example, a teenager with an obsession about being contaminated by germs may scrub his hands repeatedly (sometimes until the skin is raw and bleeding) after touching a doorknob or using the school toilets. Similarly, an adolescent who fears that she has hit someone while driving may need to retrace her route repeatedly to check that this hasn't happened.

In order to be diagnosed with obsessive-compulsive disorder, a teenager's obsessions or compulsions must cause notable distress, take more than one hour per day, or interfere significantly with his/her life. It usually begins in adolescence or early adulthood.

Generalized anxiety disorder

Generalized anxiety disorder is characterized by excessive worry and anxiety about a variety of subjects, such as school performance, social relationships, the health of significant others or world affairs. For instance, an adolescent with generalized anxiety disorder may worry much of the time about her grades, her mother's health and whether she has offended her friends in any way. Such worry will also be accompanied by additional symptoms, including restlessness, being easily fatigued, difficulty concentrating, irritability, muscle tension and sleep disturbance.

While all adolescents experience some degree of worry, the worries of a teenager with generalized anxiety disorder are far out of proportion to reality. For instance, the teenager with generalized anxiety disorder may worry excessively about failing a test although he has never received less than a satisfactory grade in that particular area, or he may believe the results of failing would be far more catastrophic than they really would be (e.g. thinking his parents would never speak to him again). Finally, adolescents with generalized anxiety disorder find it very difficult to stop the worry or to keep the thoughts from interfering with their concentration on current tasks or school assignments. Generalized anxiety disorder often begins during childhood or adolescence.

Specific phobia

An adolescent with a specific phobia experiences significant fear in response to a particular object or situation. Indeed, exposure to the feared stimulus almost always triggers an immediate anxiety response that may take the form of a situationally-bound or situationally-predisposed panic attack. There are five subtypes that describe the focus of fear in a specific phobia:

➢ *animal type* indicates a fear of animals or insects (e.g. snakes, bees);
➢ *natural environment type* is characterized by fear of natural objects or situations (e.g. thunderstorms, heights);
➢ *blood/injection/injury type* reflects fear that is cued by injury or blood or by an invasive medical procedure (e.g. surgery, receiving an injection);
➢ *situational type* indicates fear of specific situations (e.g. flying, bridges, enclosed places);
➢ *other type* is specified if the fear is cued by other stimuli (e.g. choking, vomiting, loud sounds).

A teenager with a specific phobia may avoid the situation that she fears (e.g. encountering bees), thus causing her to miss out on certain experiences (e.g. going camping with friends). Since fears are a common and often transient part of childhood and adolescence, the diagnosis should be given only if the fear has been present for at least six months and causes significant interference or distress in the teenager's life. Many specific phobias begin in childhood and continue through adolescence and into adulthood.

Part III: The three components of anxiety

The *three-component model* provides a helpful strategy for understanding, assessing and treating panic and anxiety. Rather than describing anxiety as one overarching entity, this model considers:

➢ the physical component;
➢ the cognitive component;
➢ the behavioural component.

Each of these components plays an important role in the initiation, maintenance and treatment of anxiety. Adolescents will experience these components differently, depending on the nature of their anxiety. For some, *actions* (e.g. avoiding social activities like school dances) seem to be the dominant component, causing the most distress and interference. Others may experience excessive worry in which anxious thoughts take centre stage. Adolescents with panic disorder often identify the physical domain as the central component, because of the somatic nature of many panic symptoms (e.g. racing heart, dizziness). However, in most cases, all three components are present and interact with one another to create a *cycle* of panic or anxiety.

The physical component ('what I feel')

Many teenagers who experience anxiety describe physical feelings when they feel nervous or scared. For instance, an adolescent with social phobia may feel that her heart is pounding whenever she speaks in front of the class, or a teenager with generalized anxiety disorder may experience a stomach ache along with worry. By definition, panic attacks consist of several physical sensations (e.g. shortness of breath, dizziness) that accompany feelings of intense anxiety, and adolescents with panic disorder are often particularly sensitive to and fearful of these feelings in their bodies. It is important to understand that, while these physical sensations may be uncomfortable, they are not harmful. Indeed, as described below, these feelings are simply the body's way of protecting us from danger.

The physical component of anxiety is rooted in the *fight/flight response*, an automatic reaction to danger or threat. The fight/flight response consists of immediate or short-term anxiety which facilitates either fighting or fleeing

Table 1. *Common physical sensations associated with the fight/flight response and the protective function they serve*

Sensation	Protective function
Rapid heartbeat	Allows more blood to reach various parts of the body, preparing it for action
Numbness/tingling	Blood is directed towards large muscle groups needed for action (e.g., arms, legs) and away from the extremities, causing numbness/tingling in these areas (e.g., fingers, toes). This reaction may also reduce blood loss in the event of injury
Rapid breathing	Allows the various tissues throughout the body to receive more oxygen, preparing them for action
Dizziness	A rapid increase in breathing can produce a slight, temporary reduction in blood flow to the brain which, while not dangerous, may cause sensations of dizziness, blurred vision, etc.
Sweating	Helps cool the body and prevent overheating during exertion; it may have had survival value by making the skin slippery and harder for a predator to grasp
Stomach distress	Digestion may slow down since resources are directed towards more essential processes, causing stomach upset
Muscle tension/shaking	May occur as muscles throughout the body are preparing for action
Hot flushes	May occur since activation throughout the body requires a great deal of energy
Fatigue	Often follows the fight/flight response, which requires much energy and bodily resources

danger. Anxiety served an important protective function for our ancestors by producing an automatic response that caused immediate action (i.e., attack or run) when they were confronted with danger (e.g. a wild animal). Even today, anxiety protects us in potentially dangerous situations. For instance, if a car came speeding toward someone who was leisurely crossing the street, the fight/flight response would automatically take over and the individual would run to safety.

Activation of the fight/flight response produces several physical sensations throughout the body. These sensations help prepare the body for action in a dangerous situation; however, they are often experienced as a panic attack when no real danger is present. Table 1 lists some of the most common physical sensations associated with the fight/flight response and the protective function they serve.

The cognitive component ('what I think')

Anxious thoughts are an important component of anxiety and panic. Indeed, the DSM-IV description of a panic attack includes distinct cognitive symptoms (i.e., fear of losing control or going crazy and fear of dying). The cognitive model of panic (Clark, 1986) proposes that panic attacks result from the 'catastrophic misinterpretation' of particular bodily sensations. Such catastrophic misinterpretation involves the perception of these sensations as far more dangerous than they actually are. For instance, palpitations may be interpreted as a sign of an impending heart attack, slight breathlessness may be perceived as evidence of cessation of breathing and resulting death, or shakiness may be interpreted as signalling a loss of control and insanity (Clark, 1986, p. 462).

The cognitive component of anxiety is also linked to the fight/flight response, which automatically causes attention to shift to possible signs of danger. For instance, a person who suddenly confronted a threatening bear during a hike would automatically shift attention to the bear and away from the scenic views. Adolescents experiencing difficulties with anxiety or panic often complain that they have difficulty concentrating on schoolwork or remembering assignments. While this can be frustrating to teachers, parents and the teenagers themselves, it becomes easier to understand when viewed from the perspective of the fight/flight response: attention is shifted away from everyday tasks and towards signs of potential danger or threat. When the fight/flight response occurs in the absence of danger, people often look for internal signs that something is wrong. This often results in the catastrophic misinterpretations described above (e.g. 'I must be dying, losing control or going crazy').

Some have questioned whether children and young adolescents truly experience panic attacks, and suggest that they lack the ability to make the internal, catastrophic attributions (i.e., thoughts of dying, losing control or going crazy) that characterize panic within the cognitive model (see Nelles and Barlow, 1988). A recent study challenged this notion, however, by suggesting that both children and young adolescents are capable of making such attributions in response to the physical symptoms of panic (Mattis and Ollendick, 1997a). This study included 118 children from grades 3, 6 and 9, and asked them to imagine experiencing the somatic symptoms of panic using a guided imagery exercise. Each child was then asked to complete the Panic Attributional Checklist (see Part V, Assessing adolescents with anxiety) to assess thoughts about these physical sensations. The findings revealed that, regardless of age, children and young adolescents were most likely to make internal, *non-catastrophic* interpretations of the physical sensations of panic (e.g. thoughts like 'I'd think I was worried, scared, nervous or sick'). However, some of the children at all three grade levels did make internal, *catastrophic* attributions, especially related to thoughts of dying. For example, when asked, 'What would you be thinking?' after the panic imagery, a third-grader answered, 'That I was dying or that I was going to get buried or have to go to the emergency room and get X-rayed'. Similarly, a sixth-grade child responded, 'Well, I would be thinking like I'm gonna die or I'm going to be sick in the hospital for lots of time'. Finally, a ninth-grader stated, 'that I'm hurting and I'm dying'. Further analysis of self-report questionnaires completed by the children revealed that the general tendency to make internal attributions in response to negative events (e.g. 'It's my fault that my mom got sick') as well as high *anxiety sensitivity* (i.e., the belief that anxiety or fear causes negative events such as illness, embarrassment, or additional anxiety; Reiss and McNally, 1985) were predictors of the tendency to make internal, catastrophic attributions in response to panic symptoms. In other words, these factors may set the stage for the development of panic attacks and subsequent panic disorder in children and adolescents.

The behavioural component ('what I do')

Escape and *avoidance* are the two most common behaviours associated with anxiety. Adolescents who have experienced a panic attack say that their first impulse was to get away from the situation as quickly as possible. Indeed, the fight/flight response usually makes us feel that we are trapped and need to escape. In situations where escape is impossible, this impulse may be expressed through behaviours such as fidgeting, pacing and irritability.

One reason why escape and avoidance occur so frequently is that they have the immediate, short-term effect of reducing fear and anxiety. For instance, a teenager with a specific phobia of flying knows that the anxiety he is feeling about an upcoming flight will be eliminated by simply cancelling his plane ticket. Similarly, an adolescent who experiences a panic attack before giving a speech will feel the anxiety start to abate by going to the school nurse. Of course, such behaviours serve only to increase anxiety in the long term, by sabotaging the teenager's ability to cope with the situation.

For teenagers with anxiety, the escape and avoidance responses may cause them to miss out on experiences that are a vital part of adolescence (e.g. school activities, social functions). Interestingly, adolescents with panic disorder often avoid activities that produce physical sensations similar to those that occur during a panic attack (e.g. pounding heart, breathlessness, dizziness, sweating). They may therefore refuse to go to gym class, turn down an opportunity to visit an amusement park with friends, or even refuse to watch a frightening film owing to fear of experiencing panic-like symptoms.

The cycle of panic

The cycle of panic describes the critical interaction between the physical, cognitive and behavioural components of panic and anxiety. Almost all adolescents experience physical sensations of anxiety (e.g. butterflies in the stomach), worrying thoughts ('what if I fail this final exam?') and the occasional desire to avoid aversive situations. However, it is the vicious cycle which occurs when these three components interact that sets the stage for panic attacks and anxiety disorder.

Figure 1 depicts the cycle of panic and highlights the bidirectional interaction of the three components of anxiety. This interaction creates a vicious cycle or 'snowball effect', in which physical feelings (e.g. dizziness) trigger panic thoughts (e.g. 'I'm going to faint') which exacerbate the feelings, triggering more anxious thoughts (e.g. 'I'm dying!'), and so on. Likewise, the feelings and thoughts prompt escape or avoidance (e.g. leaving the party to

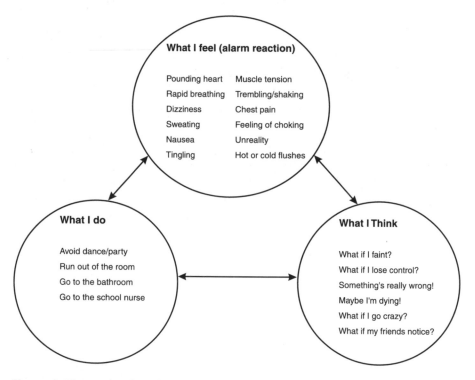

Figure 1. *The cycle of panic.*

get some fresh air or to avoid fainting in public). Ultimately, such behaviours lead to a worsening of the feelings and thoughts the next time the person is in a similar situation, since he/she is likely to attribute reduction in anxiety to escape or avoidance (e.g. 'The only reason I didn't faint the last time I felt so dizzy at a party was because I got out of there').

The cognitive model of panic (Clark, 1986) proposes that the catastrophic misinterpretation of bodily sensations plays a critical role in the vicious cycle which culminates in a panic attack. Adolescents who experience panic attacks may be *hypervigilant* to internal sensations. Such hypervigilance promotes the interaction between anxious thoughts and physical sensations, triggering the vicious cycle. In our work with teenagers, we often use the following example to illustrate this concept:

Imagine that your brain is like a watchdog that has been trained to be on the lookout for danger. When the watchdog notices anything that seems to signal danger, it sends a message to the body (which has been trained to listen carefully to the watchdog). So, when you go into a situation where you had a panic attack, the watchdog perks up and says, 'Something scary happened here before. I had better be on the lookout to make sure nothing dangerous is around.' Your body listens to this and responds by starting to prepare for the possibility of danger by making your heart beat a little faster, breathing faster, and so on. However, the watchdog, which is looking very carefully for anything that might signal danger, notices that your heart is beating faster and interprets this as a signal that something scary might happen. It sends a message to your body which says, 'Oh no! The scary feelings are starting to happen again.' The body then becomes more alarmed when it hears the watchdog say that something scary might happen, so it gets even more prepared by making the heart beat faster, creating some adrenaline, and so on. In this way, the mind and the body continue to play off each other in a sort of vicious cycle which leads to a panic attack. When these feelings continue, you may respond by having the urge to avoid or escape ('Let's get out of here!').

While the cognitive model of panic emphasizes the role played by anxious thoughts, the cycle of panic may in fact be triggered by different events in different situations and for different individuals. For instance, adolescents with panic disorder often experience this vicious cycle in response to slight physical sensations and bodily changes as a result of heightened *anxiety sensitivity* (see above). For these teenagers, even very slight changes in heart rate or slight feelings of breathlessness resulting from normal, everyday activities (e.g. gym class, drinking a caffeinated beverage) can trigger panic thoughts (e.g. 'Something's wrong with me!') which exacerbate the feelings and lead the teenager to escape from the situation. By contrast, a teenager with social phobia may experience anxious thoughts first (e.g. 'What if everyone sees me shaking when I speak in front of the class?'), followed by physical sensations (e.g. shaking, pounding heart) and a strong desire to leave the classroom.

Part IV: Understanding the causes of panic in adolescents

There is no simple explanation for why some adolescents develop panic attacks and panic disorder while others do not. As Barlow (1988) stated, 'We have only just begun to collect information on the nature of panic ... but the accumulating evidence points to a complex biopsychosocial process' (p. 209). To understand such a process, we must consider the biological, psychological and social systems of the child and adolescent, including how these different systems interact with one another and influence development. Mattis and Ollendick (1997b) proposed a pathway through which a child's temperament, patterns of attachment to significant others, and response to the stress of separation experiences might lead to the development of panic in later childhood or adolescence. This pathway is rooted in Barlow's (1988) model of the aetiology of panic, described below.

A model of the aetiology of panic

According to Barlow (1988), several vulnerabilities or risk factors are required in order for panic to develop. First, an individual must have the tendency to be *neurobiologically overreactive* to stress. In other words, some people seem to react to negative life events with what Barlow terms a 'false alarm', in which the fight/flight response is triggered unnecessarily. Since this tendency is rooted in genetics, we might expect an adolescent with this vulnerability to have a parent or other family member who also shows the tendency to be overreactive to stress.

This initial vulnerability will lead to the development of panic only under certain conditions. Specifically, it is through a process of learning over time to associate false alarms with bodily sensations that panic disorder begins to occur. As a person experiences repeated false alarms (i.e., feelings of great apprehension associated with distressing physical sensations), he/she may begin to associate the alarm reaction with the actual physical sensations (e.g. rapid heartbeat, dizziness) through the process of *conditioning*. It is through conditioning that a neutral stimulus (i.e., physical sensations) gains the ability to trigger fear after being paired with a fear-arousing stimulus (i.e., a false alarm). Once this has occurred, the individual will become extremely sensitive to somatic sensations so that even slight bodily changes (e.g. in response to exercise or temperature fluctuations) may trigger an alarm reaction or panic attack.

The model proposes that the individual must also develop *anxious apprehension* over the possibility that future false alarms or panic attacks will occur. For instance, a teenager with panic disorder will typically worry a great deal about the next panic attack and when it might occur, and may even avoid situations where it is feared one might happen. Barlow views the tendency to develop anxious apprehension as a *psychological vulnerability* that arises from developmental experiences with predictability and control.

Finally, *avoidance behaviour* may develop, depending on the person's coping skills and perceptions of safety (e.g. does a person or place exist where or with whom it is relatively safe to have a panic attack?).

Temperament, attachment and separation: implications for the development of panic

Recent reports on panic disorder have suggested that there may be a link between stressful experiences of separation in childhood and the development of panic (for review, see Mattis and Ollendick, 1997b). For instance, one study found that 65 per cent of adults with panic attacks and agoraphobia reported experiencing a traumatic separation (e.g. death of a parent, parental divorce) before the age of 15. Similarly, studies of secondary-school students have found relatively high rates of early loss experiences, including parental divorce, among teenagers reporting panic attacks. Finally, clinical studies of children and adolescents have reported an association between *separation anxiety* and panic disorder.

Utilizing Barlow's (1988) model of the aetiology of panic, Mattis and Ollendick (1997b) have suggested a pathway through which stressful separation experiences, combined with individual differences in temperament and attachment, could result in the development of panic. According to Mattis and Ollendick, children will respond to stressful separation experiences differently, depending on their *temperament* and the nature of their *attachment* relationships with significant adults. For some children, temperament serves as an initial biological vulnerability within Barlow's model, setting the stage for the possible development of panic. For instance, a newborn child who is highly reactive to negative events (e.g. cries inconsolably and is not easily soothed) may be at risk of experiencing false alarms from a very young age. Separation from a caregiver often produces immediate distress in babies and may therefore be considered a source of stress in Barlow's model. However, it is those children with *high negative reactivity* who will be most at risk of experiencing intense, prolonged distress, together with physiological arousal, when faced with the stress of separation from a loved one. An example of how a young child with such a biological vulnerability might react to separation follows:

> Amy was a three-year-old child who experienced great difficulty separating from either of her parents. As a young baby, Amy would become extremely distressed whenever she was left alone in her crib, even for very brief periods of time. Her mother described how she would cry for what seemed like hours at a time and was very difficult to comfort. As Amy got older, she would become very upset whenever her parents left to go somewhere without her. On these occasions, Amy's parents would leave her with one of her grandparents, whom Amy knew very well. However, Amy would cry inconsolably when her parents left and have great difficulty responding to her grandparents' reassurances. Amy's grandmother described Amy as appearing 'panic stricken' on these occasions, stating that she would tremble, her whole body would seem tense and her heart would be pounding.

While a child who experiences such high reactivity when faced with stressful experiences would certainly be at risk for experiencing false alarms, Barlow's model suggests that this tendency alone is not enough to produce panic. Rather, a child at risk for the development of panic disorder must begin to associate distress with physical sensations (e.g. pounding heart, trembling). Indeed, some children with high negative reactivity seem particularly sensitive to internal sensations (e.g. hunger, fatigue) while also experiencing high levels of physiological arousal (e.g. muscle tension, trembling, pounding heart) when distressed. Mattis and Ollendick (1997b) suggest that it is these children who may be most likely to associate distress with internal physical sensations after numerous stressful experiences, as described below:

> When Amy turned eight, her parents began noticing that she would seem panicky at times for no reason, even when she was with them. As her grandmother had described, Amy would seem very tense, she would tremble, her heart would be pounding and she would feel dizzy during these episodes. Over time, her mother noticed that these 'panic attacks' seemed to happen whenever Amy had been running, had become very excited, or was doing another activity that caused her heart to beat faster than usual or made her feel out of breath. After talking with a doctor, Amy's parents realized that Amy had probably learned to associate the feelings of distress she had experienced during times of stress (e.g. separation from them) with the internal sensations she had also felt at these times (e.g. trembling, pounding heart). As a result, sensations like feeling her heart beat faster while running could trigger an alarm reaction in Amy even without any source of stress. Indeed, Amy's parents remembered that she had always seemed very sensitive to internal feelings (e.g. even as a young baby she would cry a great deal when hungry or tired), probably making her more likely to associate internal sensations with distress and anxiety.

The next step in Barlow's model of panic disorder describes the development of *anxious apprehension* over the possibility of future alarms or panic attacks. This is viewed as a *psychological vulnerability* which is rooted in developmental experiences with predictability and control. Mattis and Ollendick (1997b) suggest that the child's attachment relationship with primary caregiver(s) serves as the setting within which such developmental experiences occur, and thus plays an important role in the development of psychological vulnerability.

Three *attachment categories* were described by Ainsworth (1973) based on her observations of young children in the 'Strange Situation', a laboratory procedure which reveals a child's attachment behaviour in response to minor stresses (e.g. an unfamiliar environment, introduction to a stranger, brief experiences of separation from the caregiver). Specifically, the majority of children (about 70 per cent) are classified as *securely attached*. These children use their caregivers as a secure base from which to explore the environment, separating from them to investigate toys but maintaining contact while they play (e.g. smiling at the caregiver, showing her a toy). After a brief separation, securely attached children will greet or approach the caregiver and are easily comforted by the caregiver if upset. In contrast, *insecure-avoidant* children (about 20 per cent of those studied) will separate easily but will then show avoidant behaviour when the caregiver returns (e.g. turning, looking away or moving away; ignoring the caregiver). Finally, about 10 per cent of young children are classified as *insecure-ambivalent/resistant*. These children have difficulty separating from their caregivers and show wariness in response to the unfamiliar environment. Finally, while these children show distress when separated from caregivers and approach them when they return, they also show resistant behaviour towards them (e.g. hitting, kicking) and have difficulty being comforted after the separation.

According to Mattis and Ollendick (1997b), young children who show *insecure-ambivalent/resistant* attachment behaviours may be most at risk for the development of panic. Specifically, these children will experience intense and prolonged alarm reactions with little sense of *predictability or control* since they have difficulty being soothed by their caregivers in times of stress (e.g. separation). These children may therefore learn to associate the experience of stress with negative emotions and physical sensations (e.g. racing heart) from which there is little means of escape. Over time, such children will come to view these negative feelings as frightening experiences, and may develop anxious apprehension over the possibility that they will happen again (e.g. a child may begin to worry a great deal about having 'scary feelings' when away from parents).

Anxious apprehension may also develop in the wake of traumatic separation, regardless of a child's attachment style. For instance, a parent's illness and hospitalization would be experienced by many children as a very stressful experience over which they felt little predictability or control. Even a child who previously showed secure attachment behaviour could experience high levels of distress and physiological arousal when faced with this level of stress, making that child vulnerable to the development of anxious apprehension and possible panic.

Finally, Barlow's model proposes that avoidance behaviour may develop depending on the person's coping skills and perceptions of safety. Children whose temperament leads to arousal and distress in new situations may begin to withdraw from unfamiliar people and situations as a way of reducing their distress. Mattis and Ollendick suggest that such a temperamental style will be exacerbated when a child also shows insecure attachment behaviours and has difficulty being comforted in a stressful situation. Such children are likely to feel a lack of safety and security, leading them to avoid situations as a way of coping with stress. Below is a description of a young teenager whose temperament and attachment behaviours contributed to the development of panic and avoidance:

> Jeff was a 13-year-old boy who had always been very sensitive to stress and new situations. When he was a baby, Jeff's parents recalled that he would become very distressed whenever they left him or brought him to visit a new person or place. They also reported that Jeff would seem very upset and even angry when they would return, even after a brief separation. This pattern continued as Jeff began school. Specifically, his mother reported that he would seem very nervous and would often be tearful before leaving for school in the morning, clinging to her and begging her not to leave him there. At the end of the school day, Jeff would again become distressed, clinging to his mother while also expressing anger towards her for leaving him. Jeff's parents brought him in for treatment at the beginning of the seventh grade, after he had begun to refuse to go to school entirely. Jeff's interview with the psychologist revealed that he was experiencing panic attacks at least once a week in various situations, and was avoiding going to school for fear that he would experience the 'panicky feelings' while he was there. Jeff and his parents began treatment to help Jeff cope with the panic attacks and reduce his avoidance.

In working with a child like Jeff, it is important to remember that the underlying causes of his temperamental sensitivity to stress may stem from many different sources. While temperament is usually considered biologically or genetically based, it may also be affected by experiences during pregnancy or birth (e.g. maternal stress, nutrition). Similarly, insecure attachment behaviour may result from many causes, including traumatic separation experiences as described above (e.g. chronic parental illness), temperamental factors in the child (e.g. very high levels of distress) that make that child extremely difficult to soothe, or the parents' own temperament or experiences (e.g. chronic high levels of stress) that may interfere with the developing attachment relationship.

It is important that the therapist realizes that panic disorder is the result of many factors, and that careful assessment is important to determine the nature of the disorder for each individual. The following sections review assessment strategies that may be helpful in this process, as well as ways to approach treatment with teenagers affected by panic disorder.

Part V: Assessing adolescents with panic and anxiety

One of the initial and most critical steps a therapist must take when working with an anxious teenager is to conduct a thorough, individualized assessment of the presenting concerns. This initial assessment plays an important role in guiding the treatment process, by providing detailed information on the unique characteristics of a teenager's anxiety. Furthermore, by helping the therapist understand factors contributing to the adolescent's anxiety as well as the nature of the three components (physical, cognitive, behavioural), a good assessment can pinpoint the most critical issues for treatment and allow the therapist and teenager to quickly get to work on changing the cycle of anxiety. Finally, by repeating parts of the assessment process periodically throughout treatment, as well as following treatment, the therapist, teenager and parents can identify progress and change, as well as areas still in need of work. There follows a description of some of the assessment tools that may assist a therapist in understanding the nature of an adolescent's anxiety or panic. Sources from which practitioners may obtain these instruments are listed on p. 49.

The Anxiety Disorders Interview Schedule for DSM-IV, Child Version (ADIS-IV, Child Version)

The ADIS-IV, Child Version (Silverman and Albano, 1996), is a semi-structured diagnostic interview designed to assess anxiety and related disorders (e.g. depression) in children and adolescents. During the course of the interview, an adolescent will be asked questions about her experience of anxiety across different situations. The interview is divided into sections which correspond to the various anxiety and related disorders (e.g., social phobia, panic disorder, dysthymia). Each section is introduced by one or more 'screening questions', which determine whether or not the interviewer should continue with the questions in that section. For instance, when enquiring about possible panic disorder, the interviewer asks the adolescent whether she has ever felt really scared 'out of the blue', without knowing why. If the teenager has never had such an experience, the interviewer can rule out a diagnosis of panic disorder. However, if the adolescent says she has felt really scared for no apparent reason, the interviewer will go on to assess the exact nature of this anxiety, where and how often it has occurred, the presence of panic attack symptoms (e.g. pounding heart, dizziness, fears of dying or losing control), and the degree of life interference. Based on this information, the interviewer will determine whether the teenager has panic disorder.

Following the adolescent's interview, the parents are interviewed in a similar fashion regarding their perceptions of their child's current symptoms and behaviour. To take into account potential differences between child and parent reports, the interviewer assigns two sets of diagnoses based on the separate child and parent interviews, followed by a *composite diagnosis* which includes all relevant information from both the teenager and the parents. Based on the ADIS, an adolescent may receive anywhere from zero to several diagnoses. When several diagnoses are given, usually one is considered the *principal diagnosis*, based on the extent to which it is causing interference and distress for the adolescent. To help determine the severity of each diagnosis, interviewers assign a *clinical severity rating* (CSR), ranging from 0 to 8, reflecting mild, moderate, severe, or very severe levels of distress and interference. Diagnoses receiving a CSR of 4 or above are considered clinically significant, and will often be addressed during the course of treatment. Those assigned a CSR less than 4 are considered subclinical diagnoses, because they cause limited distress and interference. These disorders should be monitored and treated if they become more severe over time.

A typical adolescent who is seeking an assessment for anxiety may receive a cluster of diagnoses at varying degrees of clinical severity, as illustrated in the following case description:

> Ben was a 15-year-old boy who was referred for an assessment by his school after he had missed classes for several weeks because of severe anxiety. During the ADIS-IV interview, Ben reported that he had begun experiencing frightening anxiety attacks two months previously, while doing a physical fitness test in gym class. He reported that he had experienced these attacks several times since, and that they were characterized by dizziness, feeling that his heart was pounding, shortness of breath and trembling. These panic attacks seemed to come 'out of the blue' and Ben had begun avoiding numerous situations for fear of having another attack. Ben and his mother also reported that he had always had anxiety about going to social events and speaking in front of others. He would become quite distressed when faced with these situations, although this social anxiety had not caused Ben to change his activities, as the panic attacks had. Finally, Ben reported a fear of heights that had begun during a family trip to the Grand Canyon three years earlier. However, while Ben reported feeling uncomfortable when in a high place, he stated that it did not cause him notable distress or interfere in his daily life.

Based on his and his mother's report on the ADIS-IV, Ben would likely receive clinical diagnoses of panic disorder with agoraphobia (CSR = 6) and of social phobia (CSR = 4), and a subclinical diagnosis of specific phobia, natural environment type – heights (CSR = 2). Panic disorder with agoraphobia would be considered Ben's principal diagnosis, given the extent to which it was causing severe distress and interfering in his life (e.g. preventing him from attending school), while social phobia would be considered a clinical diagnosis of moderate severity.

Based on this diagnostic picture, the therapist would primarily target panic disorder with agoraphobia, while attempting to reduce Ben's social anxiety as a secondary aim. Ben's subclinical specific phobia of heights could be targeted through exposure-based treatment (see Part VI, Treating adolescents with panic and anxiety) if it were to become a greater problem for Ben in the future (e.g. should he take a summer job as a guide at the Grand Canyon).

Panic Attributional Checklist

The Panic Attributional Checklist (PAC; Mattis and Ollendick, 1997a) was designed as a tool to assess children's cognitive responses to the physical symptoms of panic. This checklist, which is reproduced in Appendix 2, initially asks children or teenagers to read carefully through a scenario describing the physical sensations of panic. They are then asked to continue imagining these feelings while reading a list of 16 thoughts someone might have along with these feelings. For each thought, children are asked to indicate 'none', 'some' or 'a lot' to describe how much they would think each thought if they were having the feelings described. Of the 16 checklist items, four are positive thoughts unlikely to be associated with panic (i.e., 'I'd think I was relaxed', 'I'd think that I must be OK', 'I'd think something or someone was trying to make me relaxed', 'I'd think I was feeling that way because my room was calm and peaceful'). The remaining 12 items are divided into the following four categories representing different types of cognitive attributions a person might have in response to the physical symptoms of panic:

1. External/non-catastrophic
    'I'd think there were germs around that I had been exposed to.'
    'I'd think I was feeling that way because of the temperature or the weather.'
    'I'd think I was feeling that way because of something in the book I was reading.'

2. External/catastrophic
    'I'd think something or someone was trying to kill me.'
    'I'd think something or someone was trying to take control of my body.'
    'I'd think that something or someone was trying to make me go crazy.'

3. Internal/non-catastrophic
    'I'd think I was worried about something.'
    'I'd think I was scared or nervous.'
    'I'd think I was sick.'

4. Internal/catastrophic
    'I'd think that I must be dying.'
    'I'd think I must be losing control.'
    'I'd think I must be going crazy.'

We initially used the PAC with 118 children from grades 3, 6 and 9, and found that most children, regardless of age, tended to make internal, non-catastrophic attributions when imagining the physical feelings associated with a panic attack (Mattis and Ollendick, 1997a). However, there was a subset of children/adolescents who did tend to make internal, catastrophic attributions. According to the cognitive model of panic, such anxious thoughts would likely contribute to the cycle of panic, putting these youngsters at risk for the development of panic disorder.

The PAC can be used as a helpful tool for therapists working with adolescents with panic and anxiety since it can help the therapist pinpoint the nature of an adolescent's thoughts in response to the physical symptoms of panic. Each of the four categories described above can be scored from 3 to 9 by adding the responses to the three items within the category ('none' = 1, 'some' = 2, 'a lot' = 3). By seeing which category receives the highest score, the therapist gains a better understanding of the types of interpretations a teenager is making when faced with panic, and can incorporate this knowledge into treatment. Most adolescents with panic disorder will tend to make internal/catastrophic attributions, although they may have internal/non-catastrophic thoughts as well. The PAC can also be used by therapists as a way to assess change throughout the course of treatment (e.g. does a teenager's tendency to make internal/catastrophic attributions change following the use of cognitive strategies in treatment?).

Self-report measures of panic, anxiety and fear

There are several self-report questionnaires that may be useful in gaining a more complete understanding of an adolescent's anxiety and fears. Completing a questionnaire can help teenagers express some of the specific feelings that have been bothering them, and can be a useful tool in treatment planning as well as assessing change during and following treatment. However, it is important to remember that questionnaires can be affected by individual factors (e.g. some teenagers may exaggerate while others may downplay their anxiety). Therefore, they should always be used in conjunction with a thorough diagnostic interview, behavioural observations and information from significant others (e.g. parents, teachers).

Childhood Anxiety Sensitivity Index

The Childhood Anxiety Sensitivity Index (CASI; Silverman *et al.*, 1991) is an 18-item scale designed to assess a child or adolescent's level of anxiety sensitivity (see above). The instrument is given in Appendix 3. Anxiety sensitivity is defined as the belief that anxiety or fear causes negative events such as illness, embarrassment, or additional anxiety (Reiss and McNally, 1985). Since a high level of anxiety sensitivity may increase the aversiveness of an anxiety experience, it has been suggested that it may be related to the development of an anxiety disorder (Reiss *et al.*, 1986). In particular, individuals with high anxiety sensitivity may be more likely to develop panic disorder, since they tend to make more negative attributions about the symptoms of anxiety.

The CASI measures anxiety sensitivity in children and adolescents by presenting them with items that suggest a fear or discomfort with the experience of anxiety (e.g. 'I don't want other people to know when I feel afraid'; 'It scares me when I have trouble getting my breath'). Children are asked to endorse 'none' (1), 'some' (2), or 'a lot' (3) in response to each item, and the items are summed to obtain a total anxiety sensitivity score.

This measure can be a useful screening instrument to help identify children and teenagers who may be at risk for the development of an anxiety disorder. The CASI can also be readministered periodically throughout the course of treatment to assess reductions in a anxiety sensitivity and fear of the experience of anxiety. For instance, *interoceptive exposure* (see Part VI, Treating adolescents with panic and anxiety) is a therapeutic technique aimed specifically at reducing a person's fear of the physical sensations of anxiety. The CASI can help a therapist determine the effectiveness of interoceptive exposure for a particular teenager by indicating changes in the fear response to panic sensations.

Spence Children's Anxiety Scale

The Spence Children's Anxiety Scale (SCAS; Spence, 1997) is a 44-item measure consisting of 38 anxiety-specific items and 6 positive items (e.g. 'I am a good person') designed to reduce response bias. Children and adolescents are asked to rate how frequently they experience each symptom on a four-point scale: 'never' (0), 'sometimes' (1), 'often' (2) or 'always' (3). The ratings for the anxiety-specific items are summed to obtain a total score, with high scores indicating greater anxiety symptoms.

The SCAS also contains the following six anxiety subscales:

➤ panic/agoraphobia;
➤ separation anxiety;
➤ social phobia;
➤ physical injury fears;
➤ obsessive-compulsive;
➤ generalized anxiety.

As with other questionnaires, an adolescent's responses on the SCAS can help guide the course of treatment and indicate improvements or changes in the nature of the anxiety.

Fear Survey Schedule for Children – Revised

The Fear Survey Schedule for Children – Revised (FSSC-R; Ollendick, 1983) is an 80-item questionnaire which assesses the extent and nature of children's fear. The instrument is reproduced in Appendix 4. When completing the questionnaire, a child or adolescent is asked to rate the level of fear of various objects and situations by endorsing each item 'none' (1), 'some' (2) or 'a lot' (3). The FSSC-R includes a broad array of stimuli that children and adolescents might fear. The responses to all of the items can be added to obtain a total fear score. The FSSC-R also yields the following five factor scores, or subscales: Fear of Failure and Criticism; Fear of the Unknown; Fear of Minor Injury and Small Animals; Fear of Danger and Death; Medical Fears. A therapist can use these more specific scales to determine the nature of a teenager's most prominent fears.

Research has demonstrated a significant relationship between the FSSC-R and measures of general anxiety, which suggests that children and teenagers experiencing anxiety may also be expected to show higher levels of fear than their non-anxious peers. Indeed, a therapist should not overlook the role that fear and related behaviours (e.g. avoidance) may be playing in an adolescent's anxiety. By providing a thorough overview of an adolescent's fears, the FSSC-R can play an important role in a comprehensive assessment and treatment plan.

Multidimensional Anxiety Scale for Children

The Multidimensional Anxiety Scale for Children (MASC; March, 1997) is a 39-item questionnaire designed to assess various anxiety dimensions in children and adolescents. It provides a list of anxiety-related statements (e.g. 'I get dizzy or faint feelings', 'I worry about other people laughing at me') and asks the child or teenager to circle a number from 0 to 3 to indicate how often the statement is true for him. The MASC provides several scores and scales that can be very helpful in providing a therapist with a comprehensive understanding of a teenager's anxiety. The total score provides a measure of the overall level of anxiety, while the MASC's Anxiety Disorders Index can help differentiate children and adolescents who may have an anxiety disorder. Furthermore, the following scales allow for the identification of specific problem areas: the Physical Symptoms Scale, the Harm Avoidance Scale, the Social Anxiety Scale, and the Separation/Panic Scale. March (1997) suggests that therapists and others assessing children and teenagers be aware of patterns of scores that may indicate a particular diagnosis. For instance, a teenager with panic disorder will likely have elevated scores on the Physical Symptoms, Harm Avoidance and Separation/Panic scales.

Behavioural assessment

Direct observation of the behaviours an adolescent displays when anxious can be a critical component in understanding a teenager's experience of anxiety and appreciating the degree to which it is interfering in everyday life. In our work with teenagers, we often design behavioural approach tasks (BATs) as a way of observing a teenager's response to an anxiety-provoking situation. The primary goal of a BAT is to create a controlled situation within the therapist's office that elicits anxiety, in order to assess the degree to which the teenager is able to approach and cope with an anxiety-provoking situation. A BAT is also an opportunity to get anxiety ratings from the adolescent during a stressful situation, and often allows for *physiological assessment* (e.g. heart rate measurements), which can provide further clinical information. A BAT is often conducted before treatment, to provide diagnostic information, and again after treatment, to assess behavioural change. In designing a BAT, the tasks should be tailored to fit the teenager's anxiety profile and diagnosis. Below is a description of a sample BAT that might be used with an adolescent with panic disorder whose focus of fear revolves around the physical sensations of anxiety.

A behavioural approach task for an adolescent with panic disorder

Before beginning the BAT, explain to the adolescent that you will be meeting with her for about half an hour. You will be asking her to sit quietly for part of the time and also to do three short exercises which may cause some physical feelings (like feeling out of breath or like her heart is beating fast). Explain that you will describe and demonstrate each exercise before asking her to do it. Also explain that you will be asking her to do each exercise for a certain amount of time (e.g. one or two minutes). While you would like her to try her best to do the exercise for that amount of time, she can stop if she feels she really needs to. Explain that she should just hold up her hand to let you know she wants to stop, and you will stop the exercise.

Explain to the adolescent that every so often you will be asking her to tell you how anxious she is on a scale from 0 to 100 (where 0 is completely relaxed or not at all anxious, and 100 is as anxious as she can imagine being). This is known as a 'subjective units of distress scale' (SUDS).

Finally, all three exercises should be described and demonstrated for the teenager before asking her to perform the exercise. Use gentle cues during the exercise if you feel she is not doing the exercise correctly or completely enough to elicit physical sensations.

1. Baseline (5 minutes)

Ask the teenager to sit quietly with her eyes closed for the initial five minutes of the BAT in order to get a baseline measurement of her anxiety and heart rate, if desired. If heart rate is measured, the instrument (e.g. a pulse oximeter) should be set up and attached to the teenager just before beginning the baseline. Ask the teenager to rate her anxiety from 0 to 100 using the SUDS scale described above at the beginning and end of the baseline.

2. Hyperventilation (1 minute)

Explain and demonstrate hyperventilation for the teenager by breathing quickly and deeply, as if blowing up a balloon. Ask the teenager to do the hyperventilation exercise for one minute. Get a SUDS rating immediately before and after the exercise.

3. Recovery (2 minutes)

Ask the teenager to just sit quietly for two minutes. Get a SUDS rating after one minute and at the end of the recovery period.

4. Spin in a chair (1 minute)

Explain and demonstrate spinning in a chair (spin relatively quickly, enough to elicit noticeable dizziness). Ask the teenager to spin in the chair for one minute. Get a SUDS rating immediately before and after the exercise.

5. Recovery (2 minutes)

Ask the teenager to just sit quietly for two minutes. Get a SUDS rating after one minute and at the end of the recovery period.

6. Breathe through a straw (2 minutes)

Explain and demonstrate breathing through a thin straw (e.g. coffee stirrer or cocktail straw) with nostrils held together. Ask the teenager to breathe through the straw with her nostrils held together for two minutes. Get a SUDS rating immediately before and after the exercise.

7. Recovery (5 minutes)

Ask the teenager to just sit quietly for five minutes. Get a SUDS rating at one-minute intervals and at the end of the recovery period.

The BAT described above can help a therapist develop an appropriate treatment plan by providing important information about a teenager's behaviours and anxiety in response to certain physical sensations. For instance, a teenager who reports high levels of anxiety while spinning in a chair and who ends the task after only 20 seconds is showing high sensitivity to and avoidance of the sensations of dizziness. Using this information, the therapist could plan exercises which would help the teenager face feelings of dizziness and gradually reduce the anxiety response. This technique, known as *interoceptive exposure*, is described in the following section along with other cognitive and behavioural strategies that can be extremely helpful in treating adolescents with panic and anxiety.

Part VI: Treating adolescents with panic and anxiety

Much knowledge has been gained in recent years about the treatment of panic and other anxiety disorders in adolescents. In particular, cognitive-behavioural strategies which focus on teaching an adolescent to change anxiety-provoking thoughts and behaviours have proved very promising in reducing the distress and interference anxiety may cause in a teenager's life.

The first controlled study of the cognitive-behavioural treatment of panic disorder in adolescents was a multiple baseline design which showed the positive effects of treatment on four adolescents diagnosed with panic disorder with agoraphobia (Ollendick, 1995):

➢ Treatment began by providing the teenagers with information about the nature of panic, differences between panic and other forms of anxiety, and the treatment strategy.
➢ The second and third sessions consisted of relaxation and breathing retraining (i.e., teaching diaphragmatic breathing), with home practice of these skills assigned between the clinic sessions.
➢ Positive self-statements, cognitive coping procedures and self-instruction strategies were developed during the fourth session.
➢ Finally (fifth and subsequent sessions), the therapist introduced *in vivo* exposure through the development of a hierarchy of agoraphobic situations with the adolescent. A rationale for exposure explained that anxiety would dissipate if the teenager stayed in a feared situation rather than escaping or avoiding it. During exposure, the teenager was instructed to use the skills learned in the initial sessions (e.g. relaxation, self-instruction) to cope with anxiety.

It should be noted that *interoceptive exposure* (i.e., facing feared physical sensations associated with panic) was not an element of this particular treatment programme (see the section below on 'Panic control treatment for adolescents' for a detailed description of interoceptive exposure).

Between the fourth and fifth treatment sessions, the therapist met with the adolescent to conduct *therapist-assisted exposure*. The duration of therapist-assisted exposure ranged from 1 hour and 35 minutes to 4 hours and 10 minutes, with the therapist accompanying the adolescent to two agoraphobic situations (e.g. shopping malls). Coping strategies were rehearsed on the way to the situation, and practised during the exposure. Each exposure was terminated once the teenager was able to enter the situation and remain there for at least 15 minutes.

After therapist-assisted exposure was completed, the teenagers' mothers were instructed in the importance of exposure, and were asked to help their child arrange two 1-hour exposure trials between subsequent sessions. The remaining sessions of treatment included discussion of exposure practices and praise for progress, as well as continued rehearsal of relaxation and self-instruction strategies. Problem-solving strategies were incorporated to address and overcome difficulties. Termination of treatment occurred after a teenager had experienced an absence of panic attacks for two consecutive weeks, with total treatment duration ranging from six to nine sessions.

Ollendick (1995) reported that all four adolescents responded very well to cognitive-behavioural treatment. As described above, each teenager achieved two consecutive panic-free weeks by the end of treatment and was able to cope with agoraphobic situations that had previously been avoided. Furthermore, the adolescents reported increased self-efficacy regarding their ability to cope with panic attacks and agoraphobic situations. Notably, these reductions in panic attack frequency and agoraphobic avoidance, as well as increased self-efficacy ratings, were maintained at six-month follow-up. Decreases in anxiety sensitivity, trait anxiety, fear and depression were also reported after treatment and these persisted, for the most part, to the six-month follow-up. Finally, none of the adolescents met the criteria for panic disorder at the end of treatment or at follow-up, which suggests that cognitive-behavioural treatment can effectively reduce the occurrence of panic attacks and associated avoidance among adolescents.

Panic control treatment for adolescents

With the exception of Ollendick's (1995) study described above, there is little published research on the treatment of panic disorder in adolescents. However, a large body of research has demonstrated the efficacy of cognitive-behavioural strategies in the treatment of panic disorder in adults (e.g. Barlow *et al.*, 1989, 2000; Craske *et al.*, 1991). Panic control treatment (PCT), in particular, has shown much promise in reducing the frequency and severity of panic and associated anxiety in adults (e.g. Barlow *et al.*, 1989, 2000).

At the Center for Anxiety and Related Disorders at Boston University and at the Child Study Center at Virginia Tech, we are applying the treatment strategies of PCT to our work with adolescents. In fact, we are currently conducting a controlled research study of the treatment of panic disorder in adolescence, using a developmental adaptation of PCT for adolescents (PCT-A). The results of our treatment programme suggest that PCT-A is quite helpful for adolescents with panic disorder.

As in the adult PCT protocol, the goal of PCT-A is to address three aspects of panic attacks and general anxiety:

➤ the cognitive aspect or tendency to misinterpret physical sensations and experience anxious thoughts;
➤ the tendency to hyperventilate or over-breathe, thus creating or intensifying physical sensations of panic;
➤ the conditioned fear reactions to physical sensations.

The key components of PCT-A include:

➤ correcting misinformation about panic;
➤ breathing retraining;
➤ cognitive restructuring;
➤ interoceptive exposure.

When describing the main treatment strategies to an adolescent, we again use the cycle of panic handout (see Figure 2) and explain that the adolescent will be learning different 'tools' to target the three components of anxiety:

➤ 'Changing my breathing' is described as a tool for reducing the frequency and intensity of physical sensations;
➤ 'Being a detective' is introduced as the process of evaluating and changing anxious thoughts;
➤ 'Facing my fears' is the strategy for reducing avoidance through exposure practice.

The goal of using these tools is to break the cycle of panic by reducing physical panic sensations, anxious thoughts and avoidance, while also changing the interaction between the components. For instance, reducing physical sensations through breathing retraining will also change anxious thoughts associated with these sensations (e.g. 'I'm getting dizzier and dizzier – I'm going to faint!') and will reduce the likelihood that the adolescent will avoid the situation (e.g. leaving class to go to the nurse's office).

PCT-A is generally conducted across 11 individual sessions of psychotherapy, the content of which is outlined below.

Sessions 1 and 2
➤ The nature of anxiety and panic
➤ The three components of anxiety – physical (feeling), cognitive (thinking) and behavioural (doing)
➤ Construct fear and avoidance hierarchy

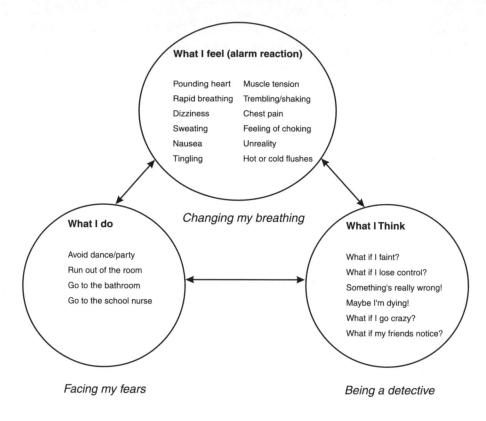

Figure 2. *The cycle of panic: treatment strategies.*

Sessions 3–5
➢ Breathing retraining
➢ Nature of cognitions (how you think now)
➢ Probability overestimation
➢ Catastrophic thinking
➢ Situational exposure

Sessions 6–8
➢ Interoceptive exposure
➢ Symptom-induction exercises
➢ Hypothesis testing ('Let's predict the future')

Sessions 9–11
➢ Continue exposure practice
➢ Naturalistic exposure (what happens in the real world)
➢ Termination

Sessions 1 and 2

The initial sessions of PCT-A are primarily psycho-educational, with a focus on describing the nature of anxiety and panic as well as the three components and their interaction. Anxiety is described as a natural, necessary and harmless part of being human. Examples of situations in which anxiety is actually helpful (e.g. anxiety would help us run to safety if a car were speeding towards us) are provided and discussed with the teenager.

Similarly, the goal of treatment is presented as not to remove all anxiety, but to remove only the anxiety that is unhelpful or unnecessary. Treatment strategies are introduced in the context of the three-component model:

➤ The adolescent is told that the physical component will be targeted by learning to slow and change breathing patterns in order to reduce the frequency and intensity of physical sensations.
➤ Treating the cognitive component involves learning to identify and challenge anxious thoughts while 'becoming a detective' (i.e., treating anxious thoughts as hypotheses, not facts, and examining the evidence for them).
➤ The behavioural component is addressed through gradual exposure to feared sensations and situations in order to change the automatic fear response to a non-fear response (thus changing the tendency to escape or avoid physical sensations and associated situations).

A *fear and avoidance hierarchy* (i.e., a rank ordering of several situations that are avoided due to fear of having a panic attack or panic sensations) is constructed individually with each adolescent and used as a guide for exposure practice throughout treatment.

Sessions 3–5

In Sessions 3–5, adolescents begin learning specific tools for coping with anxiety and panic attacks. Breathing retraining (BRT) aims to reduce the frequency and intensity of physical sensations by teaching teenagers to change from shallow, chest breathing to deeper, abdominal breathing while also slowing the rate of breathing. This is based on the observation that many individuals with panic have a tendency to over-breathe or subtly hyperventilate, thus creating physical sensations (e.g. feelings of breathlessness) which fuel the cycle of panic. Adolescents are encouraged to incorporate BRT into their everyday lives both through daily practice and by using this tool as a coping strategy when they experience anxiety.

The first step in changing anxious thoughts and cognitions associated with panic (e.g. 'I might faint!') is teaching the adolescent to identify specific self-statements that are currently part of the cycle of panic. Since many adolescents initially identify rather vague thoughts (e.g. 'I am afraid of feeling panicky'), the therapist must teach teenagers to pursue or investigate their self-statements in order to arrive at the specific thought that is fuelling the anxiety (and should therefore be the focus of cognitive restructuring). For instance:

Teenager: I am afraid of having a panic attack at school.
Therapist: What do you think would happen if you had a panic attack at school?
Teenager: It would be awful!
Therapist: What do you picture happening that would be so awful?
Teenager: I would lose control.
Therapist: What would happen if you lost control?
Teenager: I would pass out and everyone would laugh at me!

Once specific anxious thoughts are identified, strategies for challenging and changing these thoughts are taught. The concept of *probability over-estimation* is introduced as predicting that an unlikely, negative event is going to happen (e.g. 'I'm going to faint', 'I must be dying!'). A teenager who experiences such thoughts may truly believe them (much like someone playing a lottery may far overestimate the chances of winning), leading to increased fear, panic and anxiety. Treatment teaches adolescents to 'be a detective' by treating such thoughts as hypotheses or guesses rather than facts and examining the evidence for them (e.g. 'How many times has *that* happened in the past when I've panicked?'). Pie charts can be used to illustrate predicted and actual probabilities, as depicted in Figure 3.

Catastrophic thinking involves perceiving an event as catastrophic when it actually is not (e.g. 'If other people noticed that I was having a panic attack, it would be terrible and I could never face them again'). Of course, such thoughts also contribute to increased anxiety and the cycle of panic. Teenagers are taught to challenge such thoughts by imagining the worst consequence of a panic attack and then critically evaluating the actual severity and their own ability to cope. For instance:

Therapist: What is the worst possible thing that could happen if you had a panic attack at school?
Teenager: I might pass out.
Therapist: Okay. So your first thought is that you would pass out. Imagine that you did pass out. What would happen then?
Teenager: It would be horrible!
Therapist: What is it that would be so horrible?
Teenager: Everyone would laugh at me and think I was weird.
Therapist: So, what if some of the other kids laughed and thought you were weird? Does it really matter what they think?

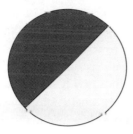

Estimated 50% chance of fainting during a panic attack   Actual 5% chance of fainting during a panic attack

Figure 3. *Pie charts illustrating predicted and actual probabilities. The therapist would first ask the teenager to estimate the chances that a certain prediction (e.g., fainting) would occur during a panic attack. The therapist would then draw a pie chart to illustrate this initial probability. For instance, the dark area of the left-hand pie chart would represent the initial belief that there is a 50% chance of fainting during a panic attack. The therapist would then challenge the probability overestimation by asking how many times the teenager had experienced a panic attack (say, 20) and how many times the teenager had actually fainted (say, 1). The right-hand pie chart would be drawn to illustrate this actual probability of 5%.*

Teenager: I guess not – but I would be so embarrassed!
Therapist: Have you ever been embarrassed before?
Teenager: Yes.
Therapist: Were you able to deal with feeling embarrassed and face the other kids again?
Teenager: Well … yes.
Therapist: Then why wouldn't you be able to handle feeling embarrassed because of a panic attack?
Teenager: It would be really uncomfortable.
Therapist: Well, yes, it may be uncomfortable, but could you deal with it? Could you handle feeling embarrassed?
Teenager: I think so.
Therapist: So, what would really be so bad about fainting?
Teenager: Nothing, really.

While teaching a teenager to challenge catastrophic thoughts, the therapist emphasizes the idea that anxiety and panic and their effects (e.g. embarrassment) are, at their worst, time-limited and manageable. Through this process, teenagers come to realize that anxiety is not catastrophic and that they have far stronger coping skills than previously imagined.

At the end of each treatment session, the therapist and the teenager choose a situation from the fear and avoidance hierarchy that the teenager can realistically practice as homework over the coming week. The purpose of these 'real-life' exposure practices is to encourage *habituation*, or a gradual reduction in the teenager's fear response to various situations. These practices also provide opportunities for the teenager to practise skills learned in treatment in order to face previously avoided situations.

The exposures are conducted in a gradual fashion, with the least feared situations practised first, then progressing to more challenging ones. For instance, a teenager who is avoiding school owing to fear of having a panic attack might initially practise going to school for a brief meeting with a teacher. Once that has been accomplished, the teenager may be ready to attend one class, then two or three, and so on until able to face an entire school day. Parents are often asked to play the role of 'coach' in these exposures, encouraging and reinforcing teenagers as they face situations from their hierarchy.

Sessions 6–8

Sessions 6 through to 8 introduce interoceptive exposure. This technique involves gradual exposure to physical sensations, with the goal of changing the automatic fear response to a non-fear response. Just as a person with a fear of heights would be encouraged to face this fear through exposure exercises (e.g. going to the top of a tall building, climbing a mountain), a teenager with panic disorder is taught to face the primary fear, namely the physical sensations of panic. By repeatedly practising exercises that produce panic-like sensations, the automatic fear response is gradually reduced.

Symptom-induction exercises are conducted in the sessions in order to identify those exercises that elicit sensations most similar to the teenager's naturally occurring panic. The following exercises are conducted, and teenagers are asked to rate the intensity of the sensations experienced, the degree of anxiety and the similarity to an actual panic attack:

➢ Shake your head from side to side for 30 seconds.
➢ Place your head between the knees for 30 seconds then lift to an upright position quickly (the teenager should experience sensations when the head is lifted).
➢ Run on the spot for 1 minute.
➢ Hold your breath for 30 seconds.
➢ Tense muscles throughout your body for 1 minute or hold a push-up position for as long as possible.
➢ Spin in a chair (relatively quickly) for 1 minute.
➢ Hyperventilate for 1 minute.
➢ Breathe through a thin straw (e.g. a coffee stirrer or cocktail straw) for 2 minutes with nostrils held together.

➤ Stare at a bright light for 1 minute and then read a short paragraph (this should be done only if depersonalization is a prominent panic-related symptom).

➤ Stare at your hand for 3 minutes (this should be done only if depersonalization is a prominent panic-related symptom).

Once the exercises have been conducted, those that elicit at least some degree of anxiety and similarity to panic are rank ordered from least to most distressing. The teenager is then asked to practise each exercise until the level of anxiety is reduced, beginning with the least anxiety-provoking and eventually progressing to the most difficult exercise. For instance, a teenager who experiences fear in response to feelings of dizziness and breathlessness may find that spinning in a chair elicits a mild degree of anxiety, while running on the spot evokes moderate fear, and hyperventilation produces the most distress. This teenager would be asked to practise (if possible) spinning in a chair until the anxiety response had diminished. Next to be practised would be running on the spot and the teenager and would finally work up to hyperventilation practice until able to face all of the exercises on the hierarchy with little anxiety.

Along with interoceptive exposure practice, hypothesis testing is introduced to encourage teenagers to face real-life situations that evoke anxiety while testing the accuracy of their predictions. In the sessions, teenagers are asked to choose an upcoming event in which they expect to feel anxious or panicky (e.g. a school dance). They are then asked to generate specific predictions that might be fuelling the cycle of anxiety (e.g. 'I will faint and have to go to the hospital'). Finally, teenagers are encouraged to participate in the event and the accuracy of the predictions are evaluated at the next session. This technique thus combines situational exposure practice and cognitive restructuring to help adolescents overcome fear, face anxiety-provoking situations and prove to themselves that anxious predictions often make a situation appear far worse than it actually is.

Sessions 9–11

The final three sessions of PCT-A focus on continuing interoceptive exposure practice, with teenagers progressing up the hierarchy once they have habituated to lower items. The ultimate goal is for adolescents to be able to perform all of the exercises that evoke sensations similar to panic (e.g. spinning in a chair, breathing through a straw) with only mild anxiety. Once this has been accomplished, the physical sensations are no longer paired with an automatic fear reaction, and the cycle of panic is broken. Teenagers are also instructed to conduct naturalistic exposures in the real world. This involves helping the teenager to identify situations that they have avoided because of the fear of physical sensations. For instance, adolescents with panic disorder may avoid gym class, amusement park rides or frightening films because of the physical sensations these activities produce (e.g. feelings of breathlessness, dizziness, pounding heart). By facing such situations, the teenager has the opportunity to practise coping strategies, such as cognitive restructuring and breathing retraining, in real-life situations while also changing the automatic fear reaction to a non-fear response.

Termination involves a review of the skills learned in treatment and encourages the adolescent to continue using these coping strategies in everyday life. The importance of continuing naturalistic and situational exposure is also emphasized. Indeed, adolescents are encouraged to become their 'own therapist' by practising skills learned in treatment and continuing to break the cycle of panic throughout their lives.

How helpful is PCT for adolescents? The case of Beth

Initial results from our Adolescent Panic Treatment Programme suggest that PCT-A is quite helpful in reducing the symptoms and distress associated with panic disorder in adolescents. Hoffman and Mattis (2000) recently reviewed the cases of two teenagers treated within our programme. One of these was Beth, whose presenting symptoms were described in Part I. Beth's initial treatment sessions were largely psycho-educational, including explanation of the symptoms of panic and the role of physical, cognitive and behavioural components in the cycle of panic. Diaphragmatic breathing and cognitive strategies were then introduced. For instance, probability overestimation was used to help Beth challenge her belief that she would faint during a panic attack. By evaluating the low frequency with which she had fainted in the past, Beth was able to replace this anxious thought with the belief that fainting was actually very unlikely during a panic attack. Beth also learned to acknowledge more realistically her ability to cope with a panic attack. Interoceptive exposure exercises (e.g. spinning in a chair, breathing through a thin straw) were initially difficult for Beth, as they elicited anxiety. However, she was able to practise these exercises successfully and experienced a reduction in her fear response to the physical symptoms of panic. Finally, Beth gradually faced the situations on her fear and avoidance hierarchy (e.g. riding an elevator, sleeping over at a friend's house). Throughout treatment, Beth's mother served as a 'coach', discussing skills learned in treatment and supporting Beth as she faced her anxiety.

One month after treatment, Beth had successfully faced all of the situations on her hierarchy and had experienced no panic attacks in the past month. She reported notable reductions in her fear and avoidance ratings of the situations on her hierarchy, as shown in Table 3.

Table 3. *Ratings on Beth's fear and avoidance hierarchy*

Feared situations	Before treatment		After treatment	
	Fear	Avoidance	Fear	Avoidance
Going to the cinema	7	8	3.5	4
Going to church	7	8	3	4
Taking the school bus	6	8	1	0
Sleeping at a friend's house	7	7	2	2
Being alone	4	5.5	2	2
Playing soccer	3	6	0	0
Being with people I'm not comfortable with	4	5	1.5	1
Being far from home	3	4	0.5	1
Going to a dance	2	3	0	0
Going to a party	2	3	0	0
Going in a lift	4	2	0	0

Note: Fear and avoidance were rated from 0 to 8 (0 = no fear/never avoids, 8 = severe fear/always avoids).

Furthermore, Beth's anxiety sensitivity score of 24 on the CASI was well within the normal range at post-treatment (at pre-treatment, Beth's score of 39 on the CASI was well above the mean for this measure).

Treating other anxiety disorders in adolescence

Cognitive-behavioural strategies can also be very helpful in the treatment of adolescents with other anxiety disorders (e.g. social phobia, specific phobia, generalized anxiety disorder, obsessive-compulsive disorder). As in the treatment of panic disorder, it is important to begin treatment with an overview of the three components of anxiety (feelings, thoughts and behaviours) and ways in which these components interact to fuel the cycle of anxiety. Skills focused on each of the components can then be taught to help break the cycle and teach the adolescent to cope effectively with anxiety. For instance, breathing and relaxation strategies can help reduce the physical sensations of anxiety, cognitive restructuring focuses on changing anxious thoughts, and exposure helps adolescents to learn to face feared situations in order to reduce their anxiety and develop coping skills. An example follows of how cognitive-behavioural strategies might be implemented in the treatment of an adolescent with social phobia:

> John, aged 15, described himself as a shy teenager who became very anxious when-ever he had to speak in front of the class or attend social functions, such as a party or school dance. In these situations, he reported that his heart would pound and he would feel 'shaky' all over. He reported thinking that others were noticing his anxiety and would laugh or make fun of him. As a result, John tried to avoid social situations as much as possible. His therapist began treatment by describing the three com-ponents of anxiety and helping John recognize how the physical sensations (e.g. heart pounding, shakiness) were affected by his anxious thoughts (e.g. 'others will laugh at me') and vice versa. John and his therapist also discussed the role of avoidance in maintaining his anxiety by preventing him from learning to cope with social situations. John then learned new methods of breathing that encouraged him to breathe deeply from his abdomen, while also slowing down his breathing and focusing on the word 'relax' while he breathed. By practising this skill, John was able to change his breathing when he was feeling anxious in order to reduce some of the 'shakiness' he usually experienced. John's therapist also taught him to challenge his anxious thoughts by 'being a detective' and treating them as hypotheses while evaluating the evidence for them. For instance, John reported that he really believed that the class would laugh at him if they noticed he was nervous during a present-ation. However, when he evaluated this thought by examining past evidence, John realized that the class had never laughed at him even though he had felt anxious many times. Eventually, John was also able to see that, even though it might be unpleasant, the world would not end and he would be able to cope if someone did laugh. John was thus able to replace his anxious thought with a more realistic thought, that 'the chances that the class will laugh are very small since it's never happened before … however, even if it did happen, I would be able to deal with it'. Finally, the therapist helped John face feared social situations from his fear and avoidance hierarchy. Beginning with the least frightening situations (e.g. calling a good friend on the telephone), John was able to confront his fears and stay in each situation until his anxiety diminished. Eventually, John was able to attend a school dance and give a large presentation in his science class. During both situations, John reported initially being quite anxious, but he remained in the situation until his anxiety diminished. Afterward, John reported that he ended up enjoying the dance and feeling very proud of his science presentation. At the end of treatment, John reported that his social anxiety was notably diminished and no longer caused extensive interference in his life.

Similar strategies to those described above may be used in the treatment of specific phobia, generalized anxiety disorder and obsessive-compulsive dis-order, although the extent to which certain skills are emphasized will depend on the nature of the disorder and the individual adolescent. For instance, the treatment of a specific fear or phobia will typically emphasize exposure to the feared object or situation (e.g. dogs, heights), while the treatment of general-ized anxiety disorder will often focus on restructuring worrying thoughts (e.g. what if I fail my finals and don't get into any good colleges?). Finally, the treatment of obsessive-compulsive disorder usually involves *exposure and response prevention* (March and Mulle, 1998), in which the teenager would be asked to face a feared situation without performing a compulsive behaviour to escape from the anxiety (e.g. teenagers with a hand-washing compulsion would be asked to get their hands dirty and then not wash them for a period of time in order to face their anxiety surrounding dirt and germs). Despite these subtle differences, the purpose of treatment is always to reduce anxiety and avoidance, increase coping skills, and enhance quality of life during the critical adolescent years.

Part VII: Working with parents

While the adolescent years are characterized by a steady progression towards independence, parents continue to play a very important role in their child's life. It is, therefore, important for the therapist to establish a positive working relationship with the parents as well as the adolescent who is experiencing anxiety. Indeed, parents can play a critical role in supporting teenagers as they face feared situations and learn to cope with anxiety in the 'real world'.

In our Adolescent Panic Treatment Programme, we provide parents with a handout at the beginning of treatment which includes information about the nature of panic disorder in adolescents, the primary treatment strategies and ways in which parents may help (Appendix 6). In addition to this handout, we ask parents to join part of the treatment sessions so that the adolescent and therapist can explain skills learned and parents can play a greater role in their child's treatment.

There are several areas that should be considered when including parents in treatment. First, it is important that parents understand the behavioural changes that accompany panic and other anxiety disorders in adolescents. In particular, parents are usually concerned about their teenager's avoidance of activities such as going to the cinema with friends or attending school events. Parents are often comforted to learn that such avoidance is quite common among adolescents with panic and anxiety, and that it can usually be overcome once the teenager begins gradually facing feared situations through exposure practice. The therapist can frame the parent's role in the exposure process as that of a compassionate 'coach' who encourages and reinforces the teenager's efforts to cope with anxiety-provoking situations.

In addition, many teenagers with panic disorder are afraid to be away from their parents, whom they regard as 'safe people' who could take care of them in the event of a panic attack. During treatment, parents should try to decrease this role and encourage their teenager to gradually face situations independently, in order to reduce the fear of being away from a parent. For instance, parents can plan to go out to dinner without the adolescent or encourage the adolescent to have a sleepover at a friend's house. The therapist, teenager and parent can work together to reduce the parent's role as a 'safe person', while encouraging the adolescent's independent coping ability when faced with anxiety.

It is also important for parents to understand the cycle of anxiety or panic and the role that it plays in maintaining their child's anxiety. Indeed, by understanding the cycle of anxiety, parents may be able to help the adolescent reverse the negative interaction between feelings, thoughts and behaviours while avoiding inadvertently contributing to the teenager's anxiety. The following case example illustrates the powerful role a parent may play in the cycle of anxiety:

> Gina was a 16-year-old who began treatment for panic disorder after experiencing numerous panic attacks in school, typically resulting in her going to the school nurse and having her mother come to get her. Gina reported that her attacks often began when she was anticipating a test or taking part in gym class – usually she would first notice that her heart was beating fast and she was having trouble breathing. After noticing these sensations, Gina would begin thinking that something was very wrong with her and would go to the nurse for 'help'. Once in the nurse's office, Gina would call her mother, who would express serious concern and rush to the school to get her. She would then take Gina to the doctor's office to be sure she was okay after 'an attack'. During the course of treatment, the therapist was able to help Gina and her mother communicate about the cycle of panic and the role each of them played in maintaining Gina's anxiety. For instance, Gina began to see how her negative interpretations of physical sensations (e.g. 'Something is very wrong with me') caused the sensations to worsen and led to a vicious cycle, resulting in a panic attack. Gina's mother was also able to understand how her response of rushing to pick up Gina from school and take her to the doctor only confirmed Gina's belief that something really was wrong. Once Gina and her mother understood the cycle of panic, they were each able to change their thoughts and behaviours in a way that actually reversed the cycle. Specifically, Gina was able to replace her anxious thoughts with more realistic ones (e.g. 'My heart beating fast is a normal reaction – it doesn't mean that something is wrong with me') and Gina's mother changed her interpretations of Gina's panic symptoms as well (i.e., she no longer believed that something was seriously wrong with her daughter). As a result, Gina's mother was able to help Gina restructure her anxious thoughts and expressed confidence in her ability to cope with the anxiety by encouraging her to return to class when she was feeling anxious. This 'teamwork' between Gina and her mother was instrumental to Gina's improvement. By the end of treatment, and with her mother's support, Gina was no longer experiencing panic attacks and was able to cope with anxiety in school.

In addition to understanding the cycle of anxiety, it is important that parents have a good comprehension of the nature of treatment and its various strategies. Parents should know that cognitive-behavioural treatment is very 'active', requiring the teenager to practise the skills frequently at home and in the real world. While the teenager should take primary responsibility for practising breathing strategies, challenging anxious thoughts and conducting exposure exercises, parental support and praise can be very helpful.

Parents should also make efforts to *model* non-anxious behaviour in their own lives, such as facing feared situations. This is particularly important because research suggests that anxiety tends to run in families, with parents of anxious adolescents more likely to experience anxiety themselves (and vice versa). The therapist should offer appropriate treatment referrals to parents who may be experiencing an anxiety disorder themselves.

Finally, the therapist should spend some time explaining interoceptive exposure to the parents so they can support their child's efforts to face feared physical sensations through exercises (e.g. breathing through a straw or spinning in a chair) and activities (e.g. running). Indeed, a family trip to an amusement park can be a wonderful final exposure practice for an adolescent with panic disorder, allowing parent and teenager to experience (and hopefully enjoy!) previously feared physical sensations.

Part VIII: Helping adolescents with anxiety: some final thoughts

Working with adolescents who are experiencing anxiety can be extremely rewarding, because the therapist is often able to witness profound positive changes as the teenager learns to cope with anxiety and lead a more fulfilling life. However, a teenager's positive response to treatment frequently requires much sensitivity on the part of the therapist to developmental issues and the unique concerns of adolescence. It is important that the therapist respects the teenager's need for autonomy and self-direction by offering appropriate guidance yet refraining from being too authoritarian. To achieve this, therapists might ask adolescents to think of them as a 'coach', while the teenager will be doing the actual practice involved in overcoming anxiety.

Adolescents often bring a perspective to the experience of panic and anxiety that is different from that of adults or younger children. For instance, teenagers with panic disorder may be less likely to express the common adult concern of having a heart attack during a panic episode. Instead, teenagers tend to express fears of fainting during a panic attack or losing control, particularly in front of friends. Indeed, social concerns are a hallmark of adolescence, reflecting the developmental task of seeking autonomy from parents and identifying with the social world outside one's family. A therapist working with a teenager must acknowledge the importance of peers and be sensitive to the impact that anxiety may be having on the teenager's friendships. Cognitive restructuring and exposure practice will often revolve around social issues and activities, whether through challenging anxious thoughts about peer relationships (e.g. 'My friends would all laugh at me if they saw me having a panic attack') or facing feared situations (e.g. sleeping at a friend's house, dating).

The therapist's sensitivity to the developmental issues and unique concerns of adolescence is critical in establishing an alliance with the teenager that will promote trust while allowing the adolescent to talk openly about anxiety. While nearly all teenagers will experience some anxiety at times, adolescents with an anxiety disorder will report significant levels of distress and interference in their daily lives. It is through the positive therapeutic relationship that the teenager can begin to learn skills for coping with anxiety, including challenging anxious thoughts, reducing physical sensations through breathing and relaxation strategies, and facing fears. Such skills empower the adolescent to reverse the cycle of anxiety and avoidance.

References

Ainsworth, M.D.S. (1973). The development of infant–mother attachment. In: B.M. Caldwell and H.N. Ricciuti (Eds), *Review of Child Development Research: Vol. 3. Child Development and Social Policy* (pp. 1–94). Chicago: University of Chicago Press.

American Psychiatric Association (1994). *Diagnostic and Statistical Manual of Mental Disorders* (4th edn). Washington, DC: APA.

Barlow, D.H. (1988). *Anxiety and Its Disorders: The Nature and Treatment of Anxiety and Panic*. New York: Guilford Press.

Barlow, D.H., Craske, M.G., Cerny, J.A. and Klosko, J.S. (1989). Behavioral treatment of panic disorder. *Behavior Therapy*, *20*, 261–282.

Barlow, D.H., Gorman, J.M., Shear, M.K. and Woods, S.W. (2000). Cognitive-behavioral therapy, imipramine, or their combination for panic disorder: a randomized controlled trial. *Journal of the American Medical Association*, *283*, 2529–2536.

Bernstein, G.A., Borchardt, C.M. and Perwien, A.R. (1996). Anxiety disorders in children and adolescents: a review of the past 10 years. *Journal of the American Academy of Child and Adolescent Psychiatry*, *35*, 1110–1119.

Clark, D.M. (1986). A cognitive approach to panic. *Behaviour Research and Therapy*, *24*, 461–470.

Craske, M.G., Brown, T.A. and Barlow, D.H. (1991). Behavioral treatment of panic disorder: a two-year follow-up. *Behavior Therapy*, *22*, 289–304.

Hoffman, E.C. and Mattis, S.G. (2000). A developmental adaptation of panic control treatment for panic disorder in adolescence. *Cognitive and Behavioral Practice*, *7*, 253–261.

King, N.J., Gullone, E., Tonge, B.J. and Ollendick, T.H. (1993). Self-reports of panic attacks and manifest anxiety in adolescents. *Behaviour Research and Therapy*, *31*, 111–116.

King, N.J., Ollendick, T.H., Mattis, S.G., Yang, B. and Tonge, B. (1996). Nonclinical panic attacks in adolescents: prevalence, symptomatology, and associated features. *Behaviour Change*, *13*, 171–183.

March, J.S. (1997). *Multidimensional Anxiety Scale for Children*. North Tonawanda, NY: Multi-Health Systems.

March, J.S. and Mulle, K. (1998). *OCD in Children and Adolescents: A Cognitive-Behavioral Treatment Manual*. New York: Guilford Press.

Mattis, S.G. and Ollendick, T.H. (1997a). Children's cognitive responses to the somatic symptoms of panic. *Journal of Abnormal Child Psychology*, *25*, 47–57.

Mattis, S.G. and Ollendick, T.H. (1997b). Panic in children and adolescents: a developmental analysis. In: T.H. Ollendick and R.J. Prinz (Eds), *Advances in Clinical Child Psychology* (vol. 19, pp. 27–74). New York: Plenum Press.

Nelles, W.B. and Barlow, D.H. (1988). Do children panic? *Clinical Psychology Review*, *8*, 359–372.

Norton, G.R., Dorward, J. and Cox, B.J. (1986). Factors associated with panic attacks in nonclinical subjects. *Behavior Therapy*, *17*, 239–252.

Ollendick, T.H. (1983). Reliability and validity of the Revised Fear Survey Schedule for Children (FSSC-R). *Behaviour Research and Therapy*, *21*, 685–692.

Ollendick, T.H. (1995). Cognitive-behavioral treatment of panic disorder with agoraphobia in adolescents: a multiple baseline design analysis. *Behavior Therapy*, *26*, 517–531.

Ollendick, T.H., Mattis, S.G. and King, N.J. (1994). Panic in children and adolescents: a review. *Journal of Child Psychology and Psychiatry*, *35*, 113–134.

Reiss, S. and McNally, R.J. (1985). The expectancy model of fear. In: S. Reiss and R.R. Bootzin (Eds), *Theoretical Issues in Behavior Therapy*. New York: Academic Press.

Reiss, S., Peterson, R.A., Gursky, D.M. and McNally, R.J. (1986). Anxiety sensitivity, anxiety frequency and the prediction of fearfulness. *Behaviour Research and Therapy*, *24*, 1–8.

Silverman, W.K. and Albano, A.M. (1996). *Anxiety Disorders Interview Schedule for DSM-IV, Child and Parent Versions*. San Antonio, TX: Psychological Corporation.

Silverman, W.K., Fleisig, W., Rabian, B. and Peterson, R.A. (1991). Childhood Anxiety Sensitivity Index. *Journal of Clinical Child Psychology*, *20*, 162–168.

Spence, S.H. (1997). Structure of anxiety symptoms among children: a confirmatory factor-analytic study. *Journal of Abnormal Psychology*, *106*, 280–297.

Further reading

Barlow, D.H. (1988). *Anxiety and Its Disorders: The Nature and Treatment of Anxiety and Panic*. New York: Guilford Press.

Davey, G.C.L. (Ed.) (1997). *Phobias: A Handbook of Theory, Research, and Treatment*. Chichester: Wiley.

King, N.J., Hamilton, D.I. and Ollendick, T.H. (Eds) (1994). *Children's Phobias: A Behavioural Perspective*. Chichester: Wiley.

Rapee, R.M., Spence, S.H., Cobham, V. and Wignall, A. (2000). *Helping Your Anxious Child: A Step-by-Step Guide for Parents*. Oakland: New Harbinger.

Sources of instruments

Anxiety Disorders Interview Schedule for DSM-IV, Child Version (ADIS-IV) may be ordered through the Psychological Corporation, 555 Academic Court, San Antonio, TX 78204-2498, USA, www.PsychCorp.com.

The Panic Attack Questionnaire (PAQ) may be obtained from Ronald A. Kleinknecht, PhD, Department of Psychology, Western Washington University, Bellingham, WA 98225, USA.

The Spence Children's Anxiety Scale (SCAS) may be obtained from Professor Susan H. Spence, School of Psychology, University of Queensland, QLD 4072, Australia, s.spence@psy.uq.edu.au.

The Multidimensional Anxiety Scale for Children (MASC) may be obtained from Multi-Health Systems Inc., 908 Niagara Falls Blvd., North Tonawanda, NY 14120-2060, USA, www.mhs.com.

Appendices

Appendix 1. Brief Screening Instrument for Panic Attacks and Panic Disorder in Adolescents

Sara G. Mattis and Thomas H. Ollendick

This checklist is intended to provide a brief overview of the DSM-IV criteria for panic attacks, panic disorder and agoraphobia in order to help the clinician screen for their possible presence in an adolescent client.

Criteria for panic attacks

Have you ever experienced an episode of intense fear or discomfort?

Yes ☐   No ☐

A. If yes, check all symptoms which occurred during the episode:

➢ palpitations/pounding heart
➢ sweating
➢ trembling or shaking
➢ sensations of shortness of breath or smothering
➢ feeling of choking
➢ chest pain or discomfort
➢ nausea or abdominal distress
➢ dizziness or light-headedness
➢ derealization or depersonalization
➢ numbness or tingling sensations
➢ chills or hot flushes
➢ fear of losing control or going crazy
➢ fear of dying

B. Did the symptoms develop abruptly and reach a peak within 10 minutes?

Yes ☐   No ☐

If the adolescent endorsed at least four symptoms and answered yes to A and B, the adolescent meets the criteria for having experienced a panic attack.

Criteria for panic disorder

A1. Have you ever experienced a panic attack (episode of intense fear or discomfort) that occurred unexpectedly or 'out of the blue'?

Yes No

A2. Have you experienced more than one unexpected panic attack?

Yes No

If yes:
A3. Has at least one of the attacks been followed by at least one month of any of the following (check all that apply):

➢ persistent concern about having additional attacks
➢ worry about the implications or consequences of the attack (e.g. losing control)
➢ a significant change in behaviour related to the attacks

B. Are the panic attacks due to the effects of a substance (e.g. medication) or medical condition (e.g. hyperthyroidism)?

Yes No

If yes to A1 and A2, together with at least one item endorsed for A3, and no to B, the adolescent meets the criteria for panic disorder. The clinician should verify this diagnosis by ensuring that the panic attacks are not better accounted for by another mental disorder (e.g. they occur exclusively upon exposure to a specific phobic situation).

Criteria for agoraphobia

A. Do you experience anxiety about being in places/situations from which escape might be difficult/embarrassing or in which help might not be available if you were to experience a panic attack or panic-like symptoms?

Yes No

If yes:
B. Do you avoid such situations, experience marked distress or anxiety about having a panic attack/panic-like symptoms when in these situations, or require the presence of a companion in order to face such places/situations?

Yes No

If yes to A and B, the adolescent meets the criteria for having experienced agoraphobia. The clinician should verify this diagnosis by ensuring that the anxiety or avoidance is not better accounted for by another mental disorder (e.g. social phobia in which avoidance is limited to social situations due to fear of embarrassment).

Appendix 2. Panic Attributional Checklist

Sara G. Mattis, PhD, and Thomas H. Ollendick, PhD

Directions: Please read the following scenario carefully, imagining that you are actually experiencing the feelings described.

> Imagine that you are sitting in your bedroom at home. Try to picture your bedroom in your mind as best you can. Imagine that you're sitting on your bed reading a book. All of a sudden, out of the blue, you start to breathe very fast. You're having difficulty catching your breath and you feel short of breath, as if you've just been running. At the same time, you feel dizzy and unsteady, as if you might faint. Your heart is beating very fast and you can feel some pain in your chest. There's a feeling of tightness in your throat and, at the same time, you feel sick to your stomach. Your hands are tingling and you feel hot. You notice that you are shaking and sweating. It's a strange feeling.

Continue imagining that you are having the feelings described. Here is a list of thoughts you might have along with these feelings. Read each statement carefully and put an X in front of the words that best describe how much you would think each of these things if you were having the feelings described above. There are no right or wrong answers – just pick the words that best describe your thoughts.

1. I'd think I was worried about something

        ____ None ____ Some ____ A lot

2. I'd think I was relaxed

        ____ None ____ Some ____ A lot

3. I'd think that I must be dying

        ____ None ____ Some ____ A lot

4. I'd think something or someone
   was trying to kill me

        ____ None ____ Some ____ A lot

5. I'd think I was scared or nervous

        ____ None ____ Some ____ A lot

6. I'd think that I must be okay

        ____ None ____ Some ____ A lot

7. I'd think there were germs around
   that I had been exposed to

        ____ None ____ Some ____ A lot

8. I'd think something or someone was
   trying to take control of my body   ____ None ____ Some ____ A lot
9. I'd think I was feeling that way because
   of the temperature or the weather   ____ None ____ Some ____ A lot
10. I'd think something or someone was
    trying to make me relaxed   ____ None ____ Some ____ A lot
11. I'd think I must be losing control

                                              ____ None ____ Some ____ A lot
12. I'd think I was sick

                                              ____ None ____ Some ____ A lot
13. I'd think I must be going crazy

                                              ____ None ____ Some ____ A lot
14. I'd think I was feeling that way because
    my room was calm and peaceful   ____ None ____ Some ____ A lot
15. I'd think I was feeling that way because of
    something in the book I was reading   ____ None ____ Some ____ A lot
16. I'd think that something or someone
    was trying to make me go crazy   ____ None ____ Some ____ A lot

Appendix 3. Childhood Anxiety Sensitivity Index

Reproduced, with permission, from Silverman *et al.* (1991)

Directions: A number of statements which boys and girls use to describe themselves are given below. Read each statement carefully and put an X in the blank in front of the words that describe you. There are no right or wrong answers. Remember, find the words that best describe you.

1. I don't want other people to know
   when I feel afraid ___None ___Some ___A lot
2. When I cannot keep my mind on my school
   work I worry that I might be going crazy ___None ___Some ___A lot
3. It scares me when I feel 'shaky'
    ___None ___Some ___A lot
4. It scares me when I feel like I am going
   to faint ___None ___Some ___A lot
5. It is important for me to stay in control
   of my feelings ___None ___Some ___A lot
6. It scares me when my heart beats fast
    ___None ___Some ___A lot
7. It embarrasses me when my stomach
   growls (makes noise) ___None ___Some ___A lot
8. It scares me when I feel like I am going
   to throw up ___None ___Some ___A lot
9. When I notice that my heart is beating fast, I worry
   that there might be something wrong with me ___None ___Some ___A lot
10. It scares me when I have trouble getting
    my breath ___None ___Some ___A lot
11. When my stomach hurts, I worry that
    I might be really sick ___None ___Some ___A lot
12. It scares me when I can't keep my mind
    on my schoolwork ___None ___Some ___A lot
13. Other kids can tell when I feel shaky
    ___None ___Some ___A lot
14. Unusual feelings in my body scare me
    ___None ___Some ___A lot
15. When I am afraid, I worry that I might
    be crazy ___None ___Some ___A lot
16. It scares me when I feel nervous
    ___None ___Some ___A lot
17. I don't like to let my feelings show
    ___None ___Some ___A lot
18. Funny feelings in my body scare me
    ___None ___Some ___A lot

Appendix 4. Fear Survey Schedule for Children – Revised

Thomas H. Ollendick

Directions: A number of statements which boys and girls use to describe the fears they have are given below. Read each carefully and put an X on the line in front of the words that describe your fear. There are no right or wrong answers. Remember, find the words which best describe how much fear you have.

1. Giving an oral report	___None	___Some	___A lot
2. Riding in the car or bus	___None	___Some	___A lot
3. Getting punished by mother	___None	___Some	___A lot
4. Lizards	___None	___Some	___A lot
5. Looking foolish	___None	___Some	___A lot
6. Ghosts or spooky things	___None	___Some	___A lot
7. Sharp objects	___None	___Some	___A lot
8. Having to go to the hospital	___None	___Some	___A lot
9. Death or dead people	___None	___Some	___A lot
10. Getting lost in a strange place	___None	___Some	___A lot
11. Snakes	___None	___Some	___A lot
12. Talking on the telephone	___None	___Some	___A lot
13. Roller coaster or carnival rides	___None	___Some	___A lot
14. Getting sick at school	___None	___Some	___A lot
15. Being sent to the head teacher	___None	___Some	___A lot
16. Riding on the train	___None	___Some	___A lot
17. Being left at home with a baby-sitter	___None	___Some	___A lot
18. Bears or wolves	___None	___Some	___A lot
19. Meeting someone for the first time	___None	___Some	___A lot
20. Bombing attacks – being invaded	___None	___Some	___A lot
21. Getting an injection from the nurse or doctor	___None	___Some	___A lot
22. Going to the dentist	___None	___Some	___A lot
23. High places like on mountains	___None	___Some	___A lot
24. Being teased	___None	___Some	___A lot
25. Spiders	___None	___Some	___A lot
26. A burglar breaking into our house	___None	___Some	___A lot
27. Flying in a plane	___None	___Some	___A lot
28. Being called on by the teacher	___None	___Some	___A lot
29. Getting poor grades	___None	___Some	___A lot
30. Bats or birds	___None	___Some	___A lot
31. My parents criticizing me	___None	___Some	___A lot
32. Guns	___None	___Some	___A lot
33. Being in a fight	___None	___Some	___A lot
34. Fire – getting burned	___None	___Some	___A lot
35. Getting a cut or injury	___None	___Some	___A lot

36. Being in a big crowd   ___None ___Some ___A lot
37. Thunderstorms   ___None ___Some ___A lot
38. Having to eat some food I don't like   ___None ___Some ___A lot
39. Cats   ___None ___Some ___A lot
40. Failing a test   ___None ___Some ___A lot
41. Being hit by a car or truck   ___None ___Some ___A lot
42. Having to go to school   ___None ___Some ___A lot
43. Playing rough games during break time   ___None ___Some ___A lot
44. Having my parents argue   ___None ___Some ___A lot
45. Dark rooms or closets   ___None ___Some ___A lot
46. Having to put on a recital   ___None ___Some ___A lot
47. Ants or beetles   ___None ___Some ___A lot
48. Being criticized by others   ___None ___Some ___A lot
49. Strange-looking people   ___None ___Some ___A lot
50. The sight of blood   ___None ___Some ___A lot
51. Going to the doctor   ___None ___Some ___A lot
52. Strange or mean looking dogs   ___None ___Some ___A lot
53. Cemeteries   ___None ___Some ___A lot
54. Getting a report card   ___None ___Some ___A lot
55. Getting a haircut   ___None ___Some ___A lot
56. Deep water or the ocean   ___None ___Some ___A lot
57. Nightmares   ___None ___Some ___A lot
58. Falling from high places   ___None ___Some ___A lot
59. Getting a shock from electricity   ___None ___Some ___A lot
60. Going to bed in the dark   ___None ___Some ___A lot
61. Getting car sick   ___None ___Some ___A lot
62. Being alone   ___None ___Some ___A lot
63. Having to wear clothes different from others   ___None ___Some ___A lot
64. Getting punished by my father   ___None ___Some ___A lot
65. Having to stay after school   ___None ___Some ___A lot
66. Making mistakes   ___None ___Some ___A lot
67. Mystery films   ___None ___Some ___A lot
68. Loud sirens   ___None ___Some ___A lot
69. Doing something new   ___None ___Some ___A lot
70. Germs or getting a serious illness   ___None ___Some ___A lot
71. Closed places   ___None ___Some ___A lot
72. Earthquakes   ___None ___Some ___A lot
73. Russia   ___None ___Some ___A lot
74. Elevators   ___None ___Some ___A lot
75. Dark places   ___None ___Some ___A lot
76. Not being able to breathe   ___None ___Some ___A lot
77. Getting a bee sting   ___None ___Some ___A lot
78. Worms or snails   ___None ___Some ___A lot
79. Rats or mice   ___None ___Some ___A lot
80. Taking a test   ___None ___Some ___A lot

Appendix 5. Treating my teenager's panic disorder: a guide for parents

Sara G. Mattis, PhD

1. What is panic disorder?

Panic attacks are sudden episodes of intense fear and physical sensations of anxiety, such as a pounding heart, dizziness and shortness of breath. While panic attacks are common among teenagers (studies have found that between 36 per cent and 63 per cent of teenagers report panic attacks!), a smaller percentage of teenagers (between 1 per cent and 5 per cent) will develop **panic disorder**. We say that a teenager has panic disorder when he/she has panic attacks that are unexpected, or seem to come from 'out of the blue'. Teenagers with panic disorder often are very concerned about having another panic attack, and they may also worry a great deal about something 'bad' happening as a result of panic ('What if I faint?'; 'Maybe something's really wrong with me').

Many teenagers with panic disorder start to make changes in their lives because of their panic attacks. One common change is to begin avoiding places where they have had a panic attack in the past or where they think it may be difficult to escape or get help if they were to have a panic attack. They may also avoid places where they worry it may be embarrassing to have a panic attack. This type of anxiety or avoidance of certain situations because of panic is called **agoraphobia**. Some teenagers with panic disorder avoid places like cinemas, public transport, staying home alone or even going to school.

Many teenagers with panic disorder have 'safe people' (often their parents!) whom they feel would be able to 'take care' of them if they had a panic attack. These teenagers may be anxious about being away from home or away from their 'safe person'. One of the reasons we feel it is so important to treat panic disorder in teenagers is that the fear of being away from parents or avoidance of certain situations can start to interfere with the teenager's life. Teenagers with panic disorder often feel that they are missing out on things like spending time with friends, going to the cinema, playing sports, or getting involved in school activities. We have seen treatment help many teenagers learn to cope with panic attacks so that the panic no longer causes as much interference in their lives.

2. Why does my teenager have panic disorder?

While we don't know exactly what causes panic disorder, we do know that panic attacks are quite common and represent part of the 'fight/flight' response that we have inherited from our distant ancestors. The main purpose of this response is to protect us by causing physiological arousal (such as increasing our rate of breathing or heart rate). This arousal helps us confront or escape from danger. Our ancestors needed this response to keep them safe during dangerous situations (like hunting in the wild) and it still protects us today (for instance, this response would help us get out of the way if a car was speeding towards us).

A panic attack occurs when the physical sensations associated with the fight/flight response occur in the absence of any real danger. Many people report having their first panic attack after a period of high stress, probably because of the emotional and physical arousal associated with stress.

While many people experience panic attacks, far fewer develop panic disorder. A key difference between people who develop panic disorder after having an initial panic attack and those who don't develop the disorder lies in the way in which we react to and interpret the physical sensations of panic. People who develop panic disorder tend to have a reaction of **fear** when they experience the physical sensations of panic. For these people, feelings like dizziness or a rapid heartbeat are scary because they are interpreted as meaning that something may be wrong. Such people tend to have **panic thoughts**, such as 'What if I faint?' or 'What if I lose control?'

Such thoughts contribute to a **cycle of panic**, in which even slight physical sensations are interpreted in a frightening way ('What if something's really wrong this time?'). Of course, such frightening thoughts serve only to increase anxiety, which then increases the physical sensations! This 'vicious cycle' between physical sensations and panic thoughts results in the continuation of panic attacks. Additionally, people with panic disorder tend to be constantly on the lookout for signs of panic, and may be alarmed by very minor (and perfectly normal!) changes in their bodies that most of us don't even notice (such as a slight increase in heart rate after physical exertion or drinking a caffeinated beverage). Such 'hyper-alertness' can trigger frightening thoughts and additional panic attacks.

The tendency to experience panic attacks and to be very sensitive to sensations of anxiety may have a genetic or biological basis, or tend to run in families (indeed, your teenager may not be the only family member who has experienced panic).

3. How will you treat my teenager's panic disorder?

A great deal of research has found cognitive-behavioural treatment to be the most effective psychological treatment for panic disorder in adults. While much less research has been done with teenagers, we believe that cognitive-behavioural treatment is the most effective psychological treatment for panic disorder in teenagers as well (indeed, we have already seen this treatment approach help many teenagers with panic disorder). Cognitive-behavioural treatment incorporates different strategies to target three areas of anxiety and panic.

First, it targets the **physical symptoms** that are associated with panic. Your teenager will learn to slow and change breathing patterns, since many people with anxiety tend to 'over-breathe' or hyperventilate in a subtle way which can increase physical sensations (like shortness of breath, dizziness, or a rapid heartbeat). Learning to slow breathing can reduce the intensity of physical sensations, while changing breathing patterns can reduce the occurrence of physical sensations.

Second, cognitive-behavioural treatment targets **panic thoughts**. Your teenager will learn to identify and challenge the misinterpretations of panic symptoms that increase anxiety and promote the cycle of panic. Challenging involves 'becoming a detective' by treating thoughts as hypotheses rather than facts, and examining the evidence for them. For instance, many teenagers with panic disorder think they will faint when they experience panic sensations. However, in reality, it is extremely rare to faint when having a panic attack. Treatment focuses on helping teenagers recognize that such panic thoughts 'play into' the cycle of panic, and to challenge such thoughts by looking at the evidence to support or refute them ('How many times have I actually fainted as a result of panic?'). Treatment also helps teenagers realistically evaluate the severity of the consequences they fear, as well as their ability to cope. For instance, even if the teenager were to faint, it would probably not be as catastrophic as he/she imagines it would be.

Finally, cognitive-behavioural treatment targets the **behaviours** related to panic, such as the tendency to escape or avoid physical sensations and situations associated with panic. Together with the therapist, your teenager will create a list of physical sensations that are part of his/her panic response. He/she will then be taught simple exercises which create these sensations (such as spinning in a chair to create the sensations of dizziness). We have found that experiencing the sensations of panic in a gradual, controlled and repeated fashion can be very effective in reducing the automatic fear reaction to these sensations (and is therefore a key to breaking the 'cycle of panic'). It is similar to riding a roller coaster or skiing for the first time. For many people, these activities are initially quite frightening, but become less scary (and perhaps even fun!) as we continue to face and practise them. Similarly, your teenager will be taught gradually to face situations that are associated with panic for the purpose of decreasing the fear reaction and increasing his/her sense of mastery and coping ability. For instance, a teenager who avoids riding the bus or going to the cinema for fear of having a panic attack will be gradually encouraged to face these situations.

4. What can I do to help?

Cognitive-behavioural treatment is very 'active' and will require your teenager to practise strategies at home and in the real world. For instance, he/she will be asked to practise new breathing strategies, challenge panic thoughts, practise exercises which create panic sensations, and face feared situations in day-to-day life. We will be asking your teenager to gradually challenge him/herself to face sensations and situations which may be initially frightening or difficult. At such times, your teenager may need your gentle encouragement and support. Sometimes it is helpful for parents to talk about times when they themselves have successfully faced challenging or frightening situations, or to discuss times when your teenager has persisted in facing a situation which was scary at first but became less frightening with continued practice (useful examples include learning to swim, ski, ride a horse). It may be helpful to your teenager if you are willing to try some of the exercises that create panic sensations (such as spinning in a chair to create dizziness, running on the spot to increase heart rate, or breathing through a straw to create feelings of breathlessness).

Finally, as we discussed above, many teenagers with panic disorder are afraid to be away from 'safe people' whom they feel could take care of them in the event of a panic attack. If you are a 'safe person' for your teenager, we will ask you gradually to decrease that role so that your teenager will learn that he/she can cope with feared situations even when you are not there.

Please talk with the therapist if you have any questions about your teenager's treatment or ways in which you can be of help. Hopefully, through treatment and with your support, your teenager can learn effective strategies for coping with panic and reducing its interference in his/her life.